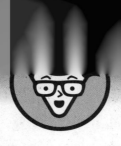

Mediterranean Lifestyle

by Amy Riolo

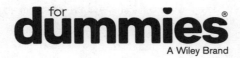

for
dummies®
A Wiley Brand

Mediterranean Lifestyle For Dummies®

Published by: **John Wiley & Sons, Inc.,** 111 River Street, Hoboken, NJ 07030-5774, www.wiley.com

Copyright © 2022 by John Wiley & Sons, Inc., Hoboken, New Jersey

Published simultaneously in Canada

For general information on our other products and services, please contact our Customer Care Department within the U.S. at 877-762-2974, outside the U.S. at 317-572-3993, or fax 317-572-4002. For technical support, please visit https://hub.wiley.com/community/support/dummies.

Wiley publishes in a variety of print and electronic formats and by print-on-demand. Some material included with standard print versions of this book may not be included in e-books or in print-on-demand. If this book refers to media such as a CD or DVD that is not included in the version you purchased, you may download this material at http://booksupport.wiley.com. For more information about Wiley products, visit www.wiley.com.

Library of Congress Control Number: 2021946525

ISBN 978-1-119-82222-6 (pbk); ISBN 978-1-119-82223-3 (ebk); ISBN 978-1-119-82224-0 (ebk)

SKY10029988_092321

Contents at a Glance

Recipes at a Glance

Fruit, Cheese, Nuts, and Desserts

Table of Contents

Introduction

Our minds normally associate the word *taste* with food. But there is so much more that we "taste" and digest each day. Our thoughts, the sights and sounds around us, the words we hear, and what we touch. At any given moment, we're inundated with either positive or negative things to focus on. After decades of focusing on the daily living styles of people in the Mediterranean region, I can honestly say that, in addition to the mouthwatering cuisine that each country has to offer, their lifestyle offers countless examples of "agreeable tastes," which you can call upon to live with both pleasure and health in mind.

The Mediterranean diet is very popular in the United States, and authors and healthcare professionals are writing and speaking on the subject all the time, but what *really* matters — more than just the food alone — are the deep roots of each of the cultural practices and daily habits that are the reasons why the diet exists in the first place.

Much of the material currently available on the Mediterranean diet discusses it within the parameters of a typical American lifestyle, not a Mediterranean one. Many doctors and cookbook authors alike are simply telling people to follow an eating plan that uses Mediterranean ingredients within the constraints of a typical American schedule. For example, they often recommend eating an Italian frittata for breakfast, a wrap with hummus and maybe some Greek ingredients for lunch, and a sensible dinner with something like salmon as a main protein. Those options *are* nutritionally sound, but culturally speaking, they're wrong. Italians eat frittata and eggs for dinner, not breakfast. Lunch is usually the biggest meal of the day in Mediterranean countries, so a simple wrap — while great on occasion — is not enough to provide the main sustenance in your day, nor does it do anything to truly celebrate the rich culinary traditions that the Mediterranean has to offer. Salmon is rich in omega-3s, but it's not native to the Mediterranean, and it has nothing to do with what the many centenarians in Ikaria and Sardinia are having for dinner. There are many other types of seafood to be had. Meals in the region are also very produce-heavy and are based on vegetables with the protein added in, not the other way around. In other words, it's not only *what* we eat but how, when, and why that matter.

With one out of every two American adults suffering from either diabetes or prediabetes and diet being the number-one killer in the United States, I'm well aware of a real need to present the Mediterranean diet not as graph chart with numbers of calories being counted, but as the true essence of the Greek word *diata,* which means lifestyle. If we truly want to live to a ripe old age while enjoying our lives with dignity and joy, we need to realize that it *is* possible and that we can do it from anywhere by embracing the traditions and customs that enable us to taste the goodness in all of life. Getting enough laughter, fresh air, sunshine, and sleep while cultivating a strong sense of community, familial ties, friendships, and support systems all work together to make the "diet" effective.

This book was created to reveal the often unspoken tenets of the Mediterranean lifestyle and the histories and philosophies of the cultures that created it, in order for you to benefit most from the Mediterranean diet. A simple eating plan, without true meaning and cultural context, can only go so far in terms of helping you to achieve your goals. When combined with other lifestyle practices, however, the Mediterranean diet can completely transform your life for the better and enable you to thrive not only at the table, but in life as well.

About This Book

Whether you're new to the Mediterranean lifestyle, you've been following the Mediterranean diet for the past 20 years, or you come from a Mediterranean country, this book will change the way you think about what you eat and how you live.

The good news is that you don't need to leave the comforts of your own home in order to benefit from this book. You don't need to buy expensive equipment or do anything radical. With simple, enjoyable strategies, you'll be able to improve not only your own life, but the lives of those around you as well.

The tips and techniques in this book can be used anywhere and are easy to implement. The recipes are delicious, authentic, and give you a wide variety of cultural inspiration to choose from. Some days are busier than others, so this book actually outlines how to fit cooking into *your* life. Most important, though, it discusses the deep-rooted misconceptions about cooking that have deprived us of one of life's greatest pleasures. Whatever your interests, lifestyle, and tastes, you'll find helpful ideas, effective plans of action, and tasty recipes that will make the Mediterranean lifestyle work for you!

This book is a reference, which means you don't have to read it from beginning to end or commit it to memory. Instead, you can dip in and out of the book as needed to find the information you need. Use the table of contents and the index to find the subjects you're looking for. If you're short on time, you can skip *sidebars* (text in gray boxes) and anything marked with the Technical Stuff icon.

When it comes to the recipes, keep in mind the following:

>> All temperatures are Fahrenheit. For conversion to Celsius, see Appendix A.

>> Vegetarian recipes are marked with the tomato icon (🍅) in the Recipes In This Chapter and Recipes in This Book lists.

>> I call for extra-virgin olive oil in many of the recipes, and there is a big difference among the types of it on the market today. It's important to choose one that has been recently pressed (within a year is best), has a low acidity rate, and has a high phenolic content. When you're shopping, search for single-estate varieties (regardless of their countries of origin), which are traceable and can provide you with that information. Throughout the book I recommend my own Amy Riolo Selections brand of extra-virgin olive oil because I've been to the land where the olives are harvested, I know the producers, and I can personally vouch for its quality (as I can the quality of the award-winning Spanish Tierra Callada olive oil, which I also recommend). If you don't have those brands on hand, any fresh, good-quality, extra-virgin olive oil will do. When you make the decision to consume a high-quality olive oil, even though it may cost a bit more, you reap many more nutritional and flavor benefits from it. Extra-virgin olive oil is considered to be not only the cooking fat of choice, but also preventive medicine and the cure to many ailments throughout the region — but if it isn't good quality, it won't have the same effects.

>> Many recipes in this book call for unrefined sea salt. Studies show that when salt is refined, the minerals that help us to metabolize sodium, such as magnesium and potassium, are stripped away. Those two nutrients are extremely beneficial to our bodies for many reasons, and many Americans fall short on their daily intake. Many supermarkets, natural food stores, and organic markets now sell unrefined sea salt for only a few dollars for a 26.5-ounce container. Look for varieties from the Mediterranean Sea, if possible, and read the label to see if it says "unrefined and minimally processed." If you prefer not to buy unrefined sea salt, feel free to use your favorite type of salt, perhaps with a lighter hand, instead.

>> If your budget allows, use organic ingredients whenever possible. But no matter what, buy the best-quality ingredients you can, from as close to where you live as possible — and enjoy them to the fullest, just as people in the Mediterranean region do.

Finally, within this book, you may note that some web addresses break across two lines of text. If you're reading this book in print and want to visit one of these web pages, simply key in the web address exactly as it's noted in the text, pretending as though the line break doesn't exist. If you're reading this as an e-book, you've got it easy — just click the web address to be taken directly to the web page.

Foolish Assumptions

In writing this book, I made a few assumptions about you, the reader:

>> You've heard about the benefits of the Mediterranean lifestyle and you want to learn what the hype is about.

>> Maybe you've been to the Mediterranean and you want to be able to enjoy the sunny aspects of the lifestyle back home.

>> You may be following the Mediterranean diet but are looking for deeper, longer-lasting results.

If any of these describe you, you've come to the right book!

Icons Used in This Book

In the margins of this book, you'll find icons meant to grab your attention and highlight key types of information. Here's a guide to what the icons mean:

TIP

The Tip icon marks important information that can save you time and money or just make your life a little easier — at least when it comes to following the Mediterranean lifestyle!

REMEMBER

You don't have to commit this book to memory, and there won't be a test on Friday, but sometimes I do tell you something so important you'll want to remember it. When I do, I use the Remember icon.

WARNING

You may encounter pitfalls along the way, and I point them out with the Warning icon, so you can deftly step around them and keep on keepin' on.

TECHNICAL STUFF

Sometimes I get into the weeds on subjects, providing a bit more information than you need in order to understand the subject at hand. When I do I use the Technical Stuff icon. You can safely skip anything marked with this icon without missing anything critical to your understanding of the text.

Beyond the Book

In addition to the material in the print or e-book you're reading right now, this product also comes with some access-anywhere goodies on the web. Be sure to check out the free online Cheat Sheet to find out why the Mediterranean lifestyle is good for you, understand how people in the Mediterranean region approach food, and more. To get the Cheat Sheet, simply go to www.dummies.com and type **Mediterranean Lifestyle For Dummies Cheat Sheet** in the Search box.

Where to Go from Here

It's time to start planning your Mediterranean lifestyle! You can start anywhere you like, but I recommend beginning by perusing the table of contents to see all the subjects this book covers. You may be tempted to dive straight into Part 4, which covers food, but I recommend reading the earlier parts first. You need to know the history and philosophy of the Mediterranean lifestyle before expecting results from the diet alone. Spending time in nature, napping, engaging in pleasurable physical activity, doing what you love, and laughing at life should all be part of your routine. Then, when you're beginning to experience some of the variety, richness, and meaning that the Mediterranean lifestyle adds to your life, you can start reading Part 4 and incorporating the food and diet aspects in your life.

Remember: A lifestyle doesn't happen in a week. If you grew up in the Mediterranean region, you would spend at least 18 years witnessing and absorbing this lifestyle every day! If you're able to understand, appreciate, and integrate *one* concept or *one* chapter every two weeks, for example, by this time next year, your life, and your health, will be totally transformed. If you have more time on your hands, and you want to experience a chapter a week, you'll have those same results in six months. A chapter a day will have you living your best Mediterranean life in less than a month. The important thing to remember is that this isn't a race — just by incorporating a few of these suggestions when it feels best to you, you'll still get pleasant and positive payoffs. Besides, to rush into anything is not the Mediterranean way.

May this book create both pleasure and good health in your life every day. Enjoy!

1
Getting Started with the Mediterranean Lifestyle

Get an overview of the concepts, strategies, and recipes that will help you live the Mediterranean lifestyle.

Learn to live the Mediterranean approach to food.

Review specific scientific research and traditions that reveal how to live better and longer by following the Mediterranean lifestyle.

Enjoy the Mediterranean lifestyle no matter where you are in the world.

Chapter **1**

Defining the Mediterranean Lifestyle

The Mediterranean lifestyle is a combination of daily living habits, customs, and traditions that have both short and long-term benefits for our health. A widely growing numbers of people are "following" the diet, but not all of them have achieved the health benefits they're aiming for. Why? Because the Mediterranean diet they're following doesn't include the essential *lifestyle* components that are key to the Mediterranean way of life. The lifestyle factors are what set people up for success.

Following a Road Map to a Health-Boosting Way of Life

Food in the Mediterranean region is much more than just fuel for physical survival. In all the various cultures of the region, preparing and enjoying food is seen as one of life's greatest pleasures. Many natives to the area view cuisine as a reason for socializing, an art form, an act of worship, a means of gift giving, a means of healing, and much more (see Chapter 2).

REMEMBER

In the United States, dieters and other health-conscious eaters tend to think of food as a foe. But in the Mediterranean region, food is a friend. Understanding this key concept is at the core of having success with the diet and lifestyle. You must embrace quality food and all the amazing ways it nourishes you in order to reap the benefits of the Mediterranean lifestyle.

Many of the recipes and culinary combinations that are popular in the Mediterranean region aren't there by accident. They were born out of millennia-old traditions in which they were considered sacred. Even ingredients that we take for granted nowadays, such as salt, lentils, and black pepper, were important forms of currency in antiquity. The Mediterranean way is to coax as much flavor, nutrition, good feelings, and healing properties as possible out of what they choose to eat.

Since the 1970s, scientists have been conducting research about the Mediterranean diet. Chapter 3 is full of research underlining the positive benefits to be had by following a Mediterranean lifestyle. It also includes expert testimonials by world-renowned doctors. If it's proof you're looking for, that chapter is for you.

You may already believe in the health benefits of the Mediterranean lifestyle but wonder how you can possibly see them in your own busy life, far away from the bright blue waters of the Mediterranean. The good news is, you can employ effective strategies to live your best life by making the Mediterranean lifestyle work for you no matter where you currently reside (see Chapter 4).

Following the Mediterranean Lifestyle

Diet and exercise alone won't provide the lasting results and rewards that the Mediterranean lifestyle has to offer. One key to the Mediterranean way of life is to see mealtimes as sacred (see Chapter 5). Having planned and pleasurable mealtimes will set you up for psychological success, which in turn affects your hormone levels and metabolism.

Another part of the Mediterranean lifestyle is laughter. Taking yourself and your life lightly, feeling good on purpose, and developing positive coping methods for adversity are all secrets to success in the Mediterranean region. Chapter 6 explains how to add a little levity to your life.

TECHNICAL STUFF

Did you know that laughing actually heals by causing the diaphragm to rhythmically contract and release the muscles until all the tension you've been holding in your solar plexus diminishes? Sometimes people even begin to laugh nervously to relieve tension after hearing bad news or during an argument. No matter where you are in the world, laughing gives you another good reason to bond socially — we're 30 percent more likely to laugh with other people than you are to laugh alone.

Finding a healthful activity — or two, or there, or four — that you can do daily will help keep you going strong well into old age. Walking vigorously for an hour a day is probably the most common form of exercise in the traditional Mediterranean lifestyle — but what is most important is that your entire body is moving and that you achieve sweat and rapid breathing for five to ten hours per week if you really want to see maximum results. Chapter 7 is full of advice about exercise and how to make it a beneficial part of your daily life.

Increased digestion, better immunity, improved mood, and reduced risk of illness are just a few of the benefits you have to look forward to by spending more time outdoors. According to one government estimate, the average American spends 90 percent of their life indoors. People in the Mediterranean, however, look for every excuse they can to be outside. Chapter 8 reveals ways to get more fresh air and explains why it's so important.

Taking naps can help you eat less and achieve an optimal weight, reduce the risk of depression, improve your mood and alertness, perform better, improve concentration, and even remove creative blocks. According to science, not all naps are created equal, and many factors impact how helpful naps can be. It's important to understand your body's own needs when trying to determine the best type of nap for you. Chapter 9 explains why naps are good for you and how to get more of them.

Considering Culture

Regardless of which Mediterranean country you spend time in, you'll recognize that daily life is a colorful mosaic of millennia-old cultural traditions, wisdom, and ingenuity, combined with modern conveniences and an ancient zest for life. Chapter 10 includes the ABCs of the Mediterranean lifestyle, a Mediterranean daily living checklist, and a brief cultural overview of each country in the region. Knowing simple yet effective strategies to call upon anytime to feel better will make the lifestyle a pleasure.

Many newcomers to the Mediterranean lifestyle are perplexed by the seemingly paradoxical tenets of some of the traditions practiced in the Mediterranean region. Many of the foods and ingredients are extremely healthful and nutrient-dense, but sugar-laden desserts like tiramisu and baklava leave some outsiders confused. When coupled with the large quantities served at feasts, it can sometimes seem like health is the *last* thing on the minds of people in the region, but that isn't true.

Chapter 11 describes why *both* feasting (practiced a few days out of the year) *and* fasting (traditionally practiced for many more days than feasting) are important benchmarks of the Mediterranean lifestyle. It also discusses the physical and spiritual implications of fasting according to the three monotheistic faiths in the region — Christianity, Islam, and Judaism.

Preparing and Eating Delicious Food

One of the biggest secrets to the Mediterranean lifestyle is the pleasure people take in food long before they eat it. In the Mediterranean region, the act of preparing a meal is a ritualistic way of not only honoring traditions and passing down heritage, but also getting more enjoyment out of the meal itself. By enjoying the process of making menus, procuring foods, shopping, growing gardens, cooking, baking, canning, or preserving, you can ensure that you're eating better-quality food while gaining meaningful insights and having fun.

Did you know that we eat less and digest food better just by *smelling* it 15 minutes prior to eating? Plus, our bodies get the same positive results when we hear our food described to us before consuming it. The sensory stimulation that our minds receive when smelling, touching, hearing about, and seeing food has as much of an impact on our bodies as tasting it does. Chapter 12 explains how you can take charge of your life by enjoying the act of preparing food. It also reveals how cooking with ancient flavor enhancers, such as herbs and aromatics, can add flavor and nutrients to your food without the fat, salt, and sugar.

In 1993, the nonprofit Oldways (www.oldwayspt.org) created the Mediterranean Diet Pyramid (see Chapter 13) in partnership with the Harvard School of Public Health and the World Health Organization as a healthier alternative to the USDA's original food pyramid. According to the pyramid, plant-based foods should make up the largest part of our diet. Fish and seafood should be eaten often. Poultry, eggs, cheese, and yogurt are important parts of the diet that should be enjoyed in moderation. Meat and sweets are at the top of the pyramid because they should be eaten the least. Chapter 13 also includes portion sizes and eating plans, and explains how to get the most out of your meals.

A well-stocked pantry can set you up for home-cooking joy and success. Chapter 14 offers a practical guide on how to do it Mediterranean-style. Having nutritious ingredients on hand at home can save you time and money. I list the cereals, pastas, grains, beans, legumes, extra-virgin olive oil, condiments, flavor enhancers, baking ingredients, and canned and jarred goods you'll want to have on hand to make cooking easier and more fun!

Chapter 15 explains how to be inspired to shop for the best food possible. Whether you're shopping at farmers markets or supermarkets, or you subscribe to a community-supported agriculture (CSA), I've got you covered. I have tips for making shopping a fun activity, creating shopping lists, and meal planning.

Eyeing Authentic Mediterranean Recipes

If you're new to the Mediterranean lifestyle, you may be overwhelmed, not knowing what to serve or when to serve it. Chapter 16 fills you in. You can find authentic Mediterranean meals, Mediterranean menus, and tips for repurposing leftovers.

TIP

Anyone embarking on the Mediterranean lifestyle needs to be able to plan menus, because there is a specific style that works in terms of flavor, seasonality, and health benefits.

When you're ready to cook, Chapters 17 through 20 are where to turn. From breakfast to small plates to main dishes to desserts, you can find a variety of recipes to take you from morning to night.

REMEMBER

It's no mistake that I saved the recipes for last. Although you may be eager to dive in to cooking, diet is only one component of the Mediterranean lifestyle. It often gets the most play in the United States, but I recommend focusing on everything else *first,* and then turning to the delicious meals. They'll be there waiting for you when you're ready to enjoy them!

Chapter **2**

Living the Mediterranean Approach to Food

D iet is important, but you'll be able to get the long-lasting, optimal health results that come with the Mediterranean lifestyle when you take culture into consideration. My grandmothers taught me, just by the way they lived, that food is the foundation that our lives, communities, and cultures are built upon. Every culture in the world offers a special selection of foods that underline not only its climate and growing seasons, but also the hopes, values, and aspirations of its culture. I often see Mediterranean diet and lifestyle books and articles that are stripped down to recipes alone. But deprived of their rich influences and histories, the recipes themselves — especially the healthful ones — seem to lack luster, even for a cookbook author like me!

When you understand the role that food plays in various Mediterranean cultures, you can make better choices. These decisions will help you to plan your daily meals better and get more mental, physical, and spiritual satisfaction from them.

In the Mediterranean region, food is a friend, not a foe. If you're interested in the Mediterranean lifestyle, understanding this key concept will set you up for success. In this chapter, I explain the concept so it sticks with you.

This chapter also reveals how food is viewed throughout the Mediterranean region — as sacred, as medicine, as charity, as diplomacy, and as philosophy and feeling. Appreciating and incorporating many of the unseen and often unexplained rituals that come into play each time certain foods are eaten can help people anywhere make more informed and fun choices. Adopting a meaningful belief about food and partaking in its customs can add life-enriching value to your daily life, which reinforces the nutritional components of your meals and has an even greater impact on your well-being. In this chapter, I explore the food and philosophical foundations of the Mediterranean lifestyle, how they came to be, and how you can reap the benefits of them anytime, anywhere.

Understanding the Role That Food Plays in Culture

In the 1950s, when American doctors first went to the Mediterranean region to do studies on the people and their habits, they went during the Lenten season. In the Southern Italian and Greek communities, particularly on the island of Crete, where the doctors conducted their research, the locals were fasting for Lent. Fasting means different things to different people throughout the region, especially in terms of eating and abstaining from food, but what the researchers came away with was skewed because of Lenten fasting. Unfortunately, they neglected to mention this subject in their reports.

In the Greek Orthodox tradition, for example, the faithful are vegan or vegetarian for 180 to 200 days of the year in order to observe religious fasts. During Lent the period of fasting means no meat, fish, or dairy (with the exception of Palm Sunday, when fish is permitted). On Saturdays and Sundays, wine and shellfish were traditionally permitted. During the pre-Christmas fasts, fish was permitted. The American researchers left Greece and wrote accounts about how you had to be a vegetarian or vegan in order to follow the Mediterranean diet, and that people enjoyed rich, long lives because they didn't eat any dairy or meat. To this day, many Mediterranean diet proponents have become vegan or vegetarian for that very reason. You can lead a very healthful life this way, but meat and dairy year-round were never intended to be given up completely. They did it as a means to adhere to their faith and culture, as many people still do today.

What was not studied at the time, but is seen as extremely important today, is the *psychological* aspects of meaningful customs and forms of spirituality. If you don't follow the Greek Orthodox faith, you can still benefit from this cultural aspect of the Mediterranean lifestyle by:

- » **Believing in the meaning behind what you eat:** Think about the spiritual and psychological motivations for eating better.

- » **Saving meat for special occasions and enjoying it when you do:** I can't imagine a Greek holiday table without lamb, goat, and other meats present.

- » **Eating dairy in moderation:** Unless you're lactose intolerant, dairy can still be part of a healthy lifestyle.

- » **Using extra-virgin olive oil as your main cooking and garnishing fat:** Entire categories of oil-based recipes are eaten in Greece and among Orthodox Christian communities during Lent.

- » **Making the majority of your meals plant based:** Fruits, vegetables nuts, grains, herbs, spices, and olives are what you should enjoy the most.

- » **Keeping in mind that the type of meat you eat matters:** Goat is much leaner than beef, for example, and lamb, ounce per ounce, offers many more nutrients than beef.

- » **Trying to ensure that the meat and dairy you consume is ethically raised and feeds on quality nutrients:** You're consuming what those animals consumed.

- » **Enjoying sheep- and goat-based dairy whenever possible:** Sheep and goat dairy products offer additional nutrients and easier digestion than cow products.

In the following sections, I explain how food is seen as a friend in the Mediterranean region and how you can adopt a pro-food approach in your own life.

Seeing food as a friend

The idea of food as a committed, loyal friend and ally is a notion that is integral to enjoying the Mediterranean lifestyle. In the United States, I often hear people say things like, "I can't even *think* about food — I'm on a diet" or "Just *looking* at that makes me fat." Statements like these reinforce the notion that food is bad for us and that food makes us fat.

In my ancestral homeland of Calabria, Italy, there is a proverb that says soups are capable of doing seven things: satisfying hunger, quenching thirst, filling the stomach, cleaning the teeth, helping you to sleep, aiding with digestion, and putting color in the cheeks. And that's just soup — imagine the proverbs they could make up about food in general!

The modern American apprehension around food (which should be reserved for unhealthful, processed foods) is hurting both our bodies and our psyches.

Food is *essential* for life. Food can cure us of many ailments and be used to keep our bodies, minds, and spirits healthy. No one gets fat or unhealthy because of food, yet one of the easiest ways to get fat is by not using food properly and not following a healthful lifestyle. The biggest enemy to the tenets of the Mediterranean diet and lifestyle is the expression "You should eat to live and not the other way around." Historically and traditionally, people in the Mediterranean region have *always* enjoyed the pleasures of the table. Even fasting times can be considered joyful and not forced abstinence. Dining well, breaking bread with loved ones, has always been the ultimate expression of the good life and a goal to aspire to. Instead of shaming this type of mentality, you can embrace it and experience enhanced well-being.

Adopting a pro-food approach

Why is so much importance placed on eating in the Mediterranean region? Well, eating is something that everyone — no matter their socioeconomic class, religion, occupation, education, or income — has the privilege or burden (depending upon your point of view) of doing every day. If you view eating as a privilege, you have the opportunity to enjoy eating every day. No matter what's going on in the world or how long your to-do list, the laws of nature give you an occasion to stop, nourish yourself, and enjoy yourself in the process. Whether you visit the westernmost areas of Southern France, the North African coast, or the Levant (the Eastern Mediterranean), you'll find that individual people and the particular cultures at large place a premium on food.

From a psychological standpoint, taking pleasure in things that we have to do anyway makes more sense than waiting for opportunities that come much less frequently to be happy. There is no reason why we need to wait for Thanksgiving to give thanks and enjoy great food. With the incentive to live better lives, we can inject a little appreciation into our daily meals.

When you're appreciative, it greatly enhances your emotional well-being. As you give thanks for food, you digest it better and absorb more of its nutrients. You don't need to have grown up in Spain, Italy, or Greece to reap the benefits of this mentality. Simply eating in a relaxed atmosphere and chewing thoroughly have big payoffs.

If you catch yourself thinking that "food is bad," here are some quick tips that will help you transform your negative thoughts into ones that will help you thrive:

>> Think about your favorite foods. Notice what you love about them. What do they provide for you? Be grateful for that.

>> Notice which foods help you feel your best. Are there foods that you truly feel good about eating?

>> Give thanks, sincerely, not only for having food, but also for the ability to grow, buy, and make it.

>> Appreciate the amount of choices that you have when it comes to eating.

>> Begin exploring the health benefits of various foods (especially those that you think you need the most).

>> Reminisce about happy times around the table.

TIP

One way you can transform your negative beliefs about food is to make meals as enjoyable as possible. It doesn't matter whether you're eating alone or in a crowd. It also doesn't matter whether you're eating a simple potato or a multi-course meal. Celebrating food helps you to make better food choices, enjoy it more, create daily pockets of happiness in your life, and enjoy a wider variety of foods, which leads to more nutritional benefits.

In order to deconstruct the task of making meals enjoyable, ask yourself the following:

>> What do you like to eat the most?

>> Who do you like to eat with?

>> When do you like to eat?

>> How do you like to eat?

>> Where do you like to eat?

Write down your answers. Set down the list and go about your life. The next day, take a few moments to go back and look at what you wrote. Carefully ponder everything you wrote and how great it makes you feel:

>> **Make note of which foods are good for you and which foods are not.** Of the foods that you love that are *not* good for you, vow to eat those only on occasion — once a week, for example, in a small portion, or once a month as a splurge. Of the foods that you like the most that *are* good for you, make a conscious effort to buy more of them, cook more with them, and enjoy them more often, maybe by discovering additional ways of preparing and eating them.

>> **Make note of who you enjoy eating with.** If you can, arrange to eat with those people more often. If you can't experience meals with them physically, try having video chats with those people while eating. At a bare minimum, you

can always imagine yourself in situations that you enjoy. Scientific research shows that simply by *envisioning* ourselves in certain situations, our bodies often respond as though we actually are in those situations, and we'll still experience health-boosting benefits.

>> **Make note of when you like to eat.** By choosing times that suit your body and schedule the best, you'll gain more out of the meal experience than if it's forced upon us.

>> **Make note of how you like to eat.** Some people prefer eating in a formal setting, and others like to eat on a blanket on the ground. Go for whatever makes *you* happy at that time, and really milk it for what it's worth. If you're sitting outside, enjoy the nature. If you're at a formal table, set the table in a way that you find to be the most attractive and pleasing.

>> **Make note of where you like to eat.** This information will help you to celebrate your food more effectively. Maybe it's a favorite table in a neighborhood cafe, a picnic spot, or a room in your home. Eating in places you like will enhance not only the experience, but also your digestion.

Celebrating Food in All Its Forms

In the Mediterranean, food is celebrated in a variety of ways, as it has been historically. In this section, I explore the sacred aspects of food in the region, how food is used to heal the body, ways in which food is considered as charity and diplomacy, as well as the philosophy behind food. I highlight ancient festivals and modern festivals and their relevance to the daily eating habits of people in the region.

Ancient pagan beliefs along with each of the three monotheistic faiths (Christianity, Islam, and Judaism), and the doctrines and religious calendars they follow, each play a significant role in the various cultures in the Mediterranean region. What may look like a simple round loaf of bread by modern standards may have had deep significance as an offering many years ago. Even mundane, more readily available daily types of bread are greatly appreciated, and adopting an attitude of gratitude plays a key role in healthful eating. Using food to heal the mind, body, and spirit is also an ancient practice that's becoming increasingly popular and helps people to celebrate food in modern times.

Food is sacred

The origins of regional Mediterranean cooking has its roots in pre–Christian times when *sagre* (ancient agricultural festivals, literally "sacred") were held in honor of various harvests in the Roman territories. The pagan gods were worshipped for abundant crops, and communities came together to prepare as many different recipes of the particular produce being honored as they could.

Fast-forward more than 2,000 years, and *sagre* are still held in Italy for various types of harvests and foods. There are festivals for as many types of traditional foods and crops as you can imagine! Everything from garlic, asparagus, and artichokes to polenta, risotto, honey, and chestnuts are celebrated at these popular community festivals. During the *sagre,* people congregate annually, usually in a particular piazza, to kick off the festivities. Vendors set up tables selling their culinary creations and local products. There are games for the children and contests for the adults. Sometimes famous chefs and celebrities are called upon to bring attention to the events. But most important, from a culinary and nutritional perspective, the *sagre* provide inspiration. Sampling fresh produce and products prepared in so many delicious ways makes it easier for people to add them into their menus at home. This, in turn, helps them to get the recommended daily amount of fruits and vegetables while enjoying themselves in the process.

In addition to the scores of festivals in Italy, other Mediterranean countries have harvest festivals as well. Some of the most well-known ones include the Egyptian date festival in the Siwa Oasis. Each June in Morocco, the city of Sefrou celebrates nature and beauty symbolized by the cherry fruit and that year's newly chosen Cherry Queen. The Sefrou Cherry Festival draws tourists from the whole nation and is on UNESCO's Representative List of the Intangible Cultural Heritage of Humanity. Greece hosts many wide-reaching and well-organized food festivals like Italy. Some of the most popular are the Aegina Pistachio Festival in late summer, the Pomegranate Festival in October, and the Pan Hellenic Feta and Pan Hellenic Mushroom Festivals in the fall.

One of the main reasons that food was viewed as sacred was because it was a form of currency in ancient times. In Ancient Egypt for example, lentils, wheat, and spices were all worth their weight in gold. Many of the Mediterranean's most splendid cities, such as Istanbul, Venice, and Cairo, were beautified by the spice trade. For these reasons, food has always been considered more than just "fuel for the body" in the region.

In Ancient Egypt, the Nile would flood twice a year, providing natural irrigation for the empire's precious crops. For that reason, huge celebrations took place honoring the rising of the river. To give thanks to what the Ancient Egyptians saw as a Nile god named Hapi, they would place on the Nile a roll of papyrus containing a prayer. Osiri was the name of the agrarian god who was cast into the Nile and returned to life. The Ancient Egyptians drew a parallel between Osiri's resurrection and the growth of wheat that was sown into the ground previously flooded by the Nile. The Ancient Egyptians also made offerings of fruits, vegetables, and flowers to show their appreciation for the Nile's rising. Dancing and singing would take place all night long, and people would drink water from the Nile.

The Egyptian love of food was even transported into the afterlife. Amulets of the son of the god Horus, named Duamutef, were created to protect the stomach of the deceased in the afterlife. From 1550 to 1070 BCE, special *faience* (earthenware) bowls were created to offer food to the Goddess Hathor, who was believed to nourish and protect the dead. The Egyptian museum in Cairo displays "food mummies" of poultry and meat, which were preserved with salt and *natron* (a local, indigenous soda from Lake Natron) and placed in tombs to nourish the dead.

When Christianity was introduced in Egypt via the preaching of Saint Mark in approximately 40 CE, the celebration of ancient festivals was discouraged by religious officials who viewed the pagan worship as a threat to the church. The festivals were forgotten about for centuries or were incorporated into the teachings of the monotheistic faiths.

Today, Judaism, Christianity, and Islam are the predominant religions in the Mediterranean region. Spirituality is viewed both as an important cultural component of each country and as a source of personal strength for its inhabitants. Many of the philosophical attitudes surrounding food stem from various religious beliefs. Natural, food-based remedies are inspired by each of the religions and followed in popular cultural. Fasting (see Chapter 11) is another spiritual concept that has a huge factor in the effectiveness of the Mediterranean lifestyle. What is eaten on holidays is extremely symbolic and representative of faith in each Mediterranean country. Sometimes, different religions eat the same foods on different occasions for various reasons.

Understanding the religious significance behind what we eat enables us to appreciate food at a deeper level and understand its role in our daily meal patterns. Egyptian falafel, for example, is a popular street food made of ground fava beans with plenty of herbs, garlic, and onions. The ingredients are among the cheapest around, and the readily available and inexpensive food is sometimes underappreciated. When I learned that the food was developed by early Coptic Christians as an alternative to meat for Lent, however, I had a whole new appreciation for it!

Further research on the subject led me to an entire volume of delicious and satisfying recipes designed specifically for Lent, a period when Orthodox Christians are vegan. Greece, Ethiopia, and other Orthodox communities in the world have special fasting dishes as well. Hailing from cultures where a premium is placed on meat and flavor, these vegan dishes are worth writing home about. I always recommend them to my vegan and vegetarian friends because they enable you to enjoy scrumptious food without meat or dairy, just has been done for centuries. The falafel is just one small example of these foods, but there are many more stories like this to share. When you learn the stories behind healthful foods, they become more appealing.

Honey, garlic, black seed, spices, herbs, and certain recipes are inspired by the religious texts. The main holy books in Mediterranean countries —the Torah, the New Testament, and the Koran — all mention foods, as well as their symbolism and health benefits. In Sunni Islam, for example, there is a collection of sayings and actions by the Prophet Mohammed called Hadith, which are followed by the faithful. The Hadith offer additional recommendations for how and when to dine healthfully, as well as what to eat (see Part 4).

Regardless of your personal spiritual beliefs, adding these beneficial elements into the diet and understanding their relevance is beneficial to both the psyche and the body.

TIP

Here are some tips for incorporating the sacred aspect of food in your daily life:

>> Determine whether there are any healthful foods or recipes that are special to you for significant reasons, and incorporate them into your life as much as possible.

>> Spend some time researching the health benefits of your favorite ingredients, and find ways to enjoy more of them.

>> If you're prone to or experiencing a particular ailment, find out which herb, spice, or ingredient is most beneficial to healing the condition and eat more of it.

>> Infuse your daily life with more meaningful foods in whatever way gives you the most pleasure.

Incorporating these concepts will add Mediterranean-style meaning to your meals and help the foods you eat to sooth your psyche, as well as satisfy your palate.

Food is medicine

Foods have been used to heal the body for millennia, but modern culture doesn't always take advantage of food's healing properties. Diet is the number-one killer in the United States, and many people are looking for new ways to not only heal themselves, but also prevent illness, while enjoying their food at the same time. *Culinary medicine* (the combination of the art of cooking and eating with science, nutrition, and medicine) is gaining increasing popularity all around the world. It's greatly needed, especially in the United States, where poor diet and physical activity combined are the leading cause of death.

Culinary medicine and the Mediterranean region go hand in hand. Hippocrates used to prescribe foods such as olive oil to cure gastritis and ulcers. Although modern medicine is readily available and used in the region today, most people automatically start looking for foods to cure and prevent illness before they even *think* about medicine. For example, if you happen to be in Lebanon, and you have a cough or congestion, you'll be served *zait wa zaatar* (olive oil and a dried spice mixture made up of wild thyme). Thyme has been scientifically proven to be an excellent cough suppressant (a chemical derivative of it is used as an ingredient in modern cough syrups), and good-quality olive oil helps to increase the absorption and potency of thyme while also adding powerful antioxidant and anti-inflammatory benefits to the mix. Many Italians eat fennel after a large meal or drink fennel-infused digestifs to help with digestion. In Egypt, you may be served anise tea to help you sleep or a hibiscus-infused drink to lower blood pressure.

REMEMBER

Each natural food has a specific nutritional benefit; when the food is eaten properly, it can help prevent and cure disease. Powerful nutrients in many foods can help not only the body, but the mind and spirit. Mediterranean regional cooking is full of what I like to call "eat me first" foods — broccoli and dark leafy greens like purslane, dandelion greens, Swiss chard, kale, collards, and spinach along with fresh fish, for example, combined with other nutrient-dense plant-based ingredients. Eating a steady diet of these types of foods (also referred to as those coming from the "gardens of longevity") will help to ensure that, from a consumption standpoint, you're maximizing your nutrition. Overall, the traditional Mediterranean diet (the food that was being consumed on a daily basis in pre-1960 Greece and surrounding countries) is beneficial to optimal mental, physical, and spiritual health. The Mediterranean diet itself has been shown to help the mind, brain, and mood.

Whether you're dealing with or you want to prevent depression, anxiety, memory loss, or brain injuries, foods that have an anti-inflammatory effect can be very helpful. The bioactive nutrients in broccoli, for example, can switch on DNA to activate the powerful antioxidants, detoxify enzymes, and other compounds needed to create powerful changes in well-being. Foods rich in omega-3s such as sardines, salmon, eggs, flaxseed, purslane, and walnuts, are all powerful brain health boosters. The antioxidants in extra-virgin olive oil reduce the risk of dementia, clear away brain toxins, and reduce plaque formation in the brain and arteries.

Health can be greatly improved by following the Mediterranean diet in general. But culinary medicine goes a few steps beyond "good for you" food to ensure that you're eating the best foods that *your* body needs, giving you the most nutritional bang for your buck.

That said, there are specific foods that contain certain nutrients that our bodies need at certain times. Understanding the needs of our individual bodies at various times can be extremely beneficial in determining our culinary medicine needs. Someone who is dealing with a particular illness, for example, can eat certain foods to help them to transform their illness.

Inulin-rich foods such as Greek yogurt, basil, extra-virgin olive oil, dark chocolate, and good-quality balsamic vinegar (with no sugar or preservatives added) can help balance blood-sugar levels in people with diabetes. In addition, onions help to clear away toxins in the cells, garlic is a natural antibiotic, and cloves have antiseptic properties. The lists of foods that help specific conditions is long enough to fill an entire book, but just knowing that food has this power is a step in the right direction. The recipes and food combinations in this book will help you get started putting these principles to good use.

Foods that enhance our spiritual well-being come in three categories in the Mediterranean region:

>> **Foods that are pleasurable and that you enjoy eating the most:** This category may include a special sweet treat, a food that you're nostalgic about from your childhood, or a gourmet treat that may be more of a splurge in terms of fat and calories but that you really enjoy and look forward to eating. These foods are ones that should be saved for holidays and large family gatherings.

>> **Foods that have the power to elevate your mood:** The omega-3s in seafood are believed to do that, but it's the aroma of citrus (orange, lemon, and bergamot) that's most widely used to make people's days brighter. *Assir limon,* a frothy lemonade, is often served to nervous people to elevate their mood in Egypt. Freshly squeezed orange juice is served at breakfast in many countries, and the enchanting aroma from the orange blossom itself is wafted everywhere to lift spirits in Morocco. In my ancestral homeland of Calabria, bergamot (the signature aroma in Earl Grey tea and many fragrances) grows. We use bergamot in everything from jam to cologne to an essential oil that can be burned to release an elevating scent. Recently, it has also been proven to have excellent benefits on glucose and cholesterol. Turmeric is an ancient spice that has great mood-boosting ingredients (especially when made into a cool drink with citrus juice and honey); some people claim it's more potent than Prozac. Rosemary helps stimulate memory and brain activity; it's even rubbed into the scalp to stimulate hair growth.

>> **Religious-based foods to elevate the spirit:** In addition to benefiting from the nutrition of the food itself, many people in the Mediterranean region use spiritual practices to further benefit from their food. Many say blessings on specific dishes in order to receive more benefit from them. The Kosher dietary laws in many Jewish households, along with the Halal requirements in many Muslim ones, and the rules of fasting Christians, add additional layers of spiritual benefits to those who believe in the meaning behind them. Eating certain foods or eating foods in a certain way for a higher purpose has emotionally and mentally satisfying rewards. Be grateful for food, savor every bite, and eat as if food is a means of honoring the life force within us, and the life force itself will set you up for success at the table, regardless of your personal creed or the actual food that's on the table.

CREATING YOUR MOOD WITH FOOD

Modern Western medical advice suggests that we not let our moods control what we eat. We're supposed to eat healthfully, and perhaps the same types of foods, no matter what's going on with our emotions. I've never found that to be a particularly healthful strategy, and it's definitely not how things are done in the Mediterranean region. Whether you grow up in the South of France, Greece, or the mountains of Lebanon, you learn that emotions are important to acknowledge and that you can use foods in specific ways either to create or help cope with certain emotions.

I remember the first time I was working in Egypt. One of my coworkers walked in and, instead of saying, "How are you?," he said, "What is your mood?" I became extremely defensive and thought that he was implying that something was wrong or that I had an attitude problem by inquiring about my mood. He later explained (and others confirmed), that this is often a question asked among close friends. By asking each other what mood we are in, he explained, we can better interact with each other. If someone is sad, you can cheer them up; if they're happy, you can rejoice with them.

From a culinary perspective, that made a lot of sense to me. I grew up learning how to use food to create people's moods. As the family cook from a young age, I saw firsthand the effect that eating certain foods had on my family. Creamy foods, for example, usually evoke a sense of care and comfort, while crunchy foods help us fill a craving for adventure and fun.

The term *comfort food* has an indirect double meaning of "unhealthy" in the United States. Many people associate comfort food with junk food or sugary, high-fat desserts, but that isn't always the case. A simple rice pudding made with milk, rice, vanilla, citrus zest, and a tiny bit of sugar can be soothing. In Egypt, that's a typical breakfast, often eaten instead of cereal. Creamy mashed potatoes seasoned with extra-virgin olive oil and herbs instead of loads of butter and salt can give that same wonderful mouth feel and satisfaction you desire.

I also really like to make people (or myself) foods from my youth when I'm stressed. Recipes that evoke happy memories can lift the mood in a hurry. When I do this for friends, they're usually pleasantly surprised at the culinary trip back in time to their childhoods. One such recipe that always makes me feel better is spaghetti with garlic, chilies, and extra-virgin olive oil. I've fought off everything from melancholy to migraines and muscle pain with just one serving. Scientifically speaking, this is because the extra-virgin olive oil, garlic, and chilies are all anti-inflammatory ingredients and cause a reaction that helps the body to feel less pain. The carbohydrates give an energy boost, which also enables you to feel better. In addition, the combination of flavors and textures, which signify well-being to the psyche, make any day seem brighter.

Trouble comes in when we rely exclusively on foods to correct or deal with negative emotions. In our modern society, I find that sometimes people don't even distinguish the difference between positive and negative emotions — they just lump all of them into the same unwanted category. In the Mediterranean region, the goal is to feel as many of the positive emotions as much as possible. So, if a "dose" of spaghetti all'aglio e olio or your grandmother's rice pudding recipe doesn't improve your mood, it's time to call upon the other lifestyle components to help correct them.

Culinary medicine can be a helpful way to boost your mood when you're depressed or calm your nerves when you're overly excited. Magnesium in dark, leafy green vegetables, omega-3s in sardines, mackerel, and flax-seeds; and vitamin C in citrus such as orange, lemon, and bergamot have all been proven to elevate the mood. Smelling the aroma of citrus alone — without even eating it — can have a positive effect on your overall outlook.

Food is charity

Giving food as charity, or as a gift in general, has been done all over the world since the beginning of time. In modern times, it may seem odd that people would prefer to give and receive food than money. But in the Mediterranean region, people pay attention to what kind of food they give away, whether as a present or as a form of charity. In the Mediterranean, it is customary in many cultures to give away or donate food that people enjoy and that is meaningful to them. These notions underscore the importance of community in the region.

In Muslim countries in the Mediterranean and elsewhere, whenever someone is grateful for a blessing, it's customary to slaughter an animal and distribute the meat to neighbors and the needy. In Morocco, women often gather to make homemade couscous, the local staple, to distribute to the less fortunate. Throughout the region, it's considered rude to eat something and not offer it to those around you, so when large celebrations take place, people think about what they're giving to the community.

Several dishes — such as wheat puddings when celebrating a birth, celebratory dishes at weddings, and sweets on special occasions — are often shared with more neighbors and community members than would typically happen in the United States. In Naples, Italy, for example, espresso is taken very seriously, and people even give espresso to the poor. In Naples, there is a tradition called a *caffe sospeso* (suspended coffee). Someone can enter a bar or cafe and order one in order to pay it forward for a guest who can't pay for their own.

The annual Cous Cous Fest in San Vito Lo Capo, Italy offers a ten-day extravaganza dedicated entirely to couscous and has become known internationally as a Festival of Food and Cultural Integration. The festival hosts renowned chefs from more than ten countries where couscous is popular and offers more than 30 couscous recipes. Free nightly concerts include some of the world's most beloved artists — also from couscous-loving cultures. The festival celebrates couscous as a symbol of peace and unity among the peoples of the world. In addition, the event gives voice to the refugee crisis in the region while promoting typical foods of Sicily, the host country.

Food is diplomacy

People began extending olive branches as a symbol of peace in antiquity because olive trees only bore fruit after being planted for 20 years. This meant that olive trees weren't planted in unpeaceful places. As a result, olive branches became synonymous with peace around the world. Olive oil, as an ingredient, connects the Mediterranean region with the world at large on a daily basis, while enhancing our health.

The Couscous Fest (see the preceding section) is the perfect example of how food can be used to build a culinary bridge. In Nomadic times, tribes who were traveling to new territories would stop along their way. They would offer the seminomadic tribes that they encountered news of climatic events and conquering tribes and other dangers to look out for in exchange for food and shelter. Although *culinary diplomacy* is a more modern term, its tenets started with those tribes, and in the Mediterranean region we see it on display constantly.

Whether people are trying to improve relations in their private or professional lives or with other communities, food is a direct and powerful form of diplomacy. Historically speaking, there is evidence, for example, of Egyptian Sultans giving trays of fish and sweet doughnuts to Christian clerics for Christmas. This shows that the giver gave something that was significant to the recipient (fish were a delicacy for Christmas at the time, as were the doughnuts). In the Muslim faith, it's required to pay a certain amount of charity during Ramadan in order for the month's worth of fasting and good deeds to be accepted by the divine. In the 10th century, Egypt's rulers would distribute *kahk al'eid* (traditional Eid cookies, stuffed with gold) to the poor. Nowadays those cookies are still eaten for the holiday, but stuffed with edible fillings reminiscent of the gold.

Hospitality is paramount in the Mediterranean lifestyle. Regardless of the specific country or culture people come from, people in the region derive a strong sense of pride and purpose by being able to cook and care for others. Without trying to do so, the acts of hospitality help build community whether it's on a large or small scale. The English word for hospitality comes from the Latin *hospitem*, which was used during a time when the act of receiving a guest was an honor.

To this day, in the Mediterranean region, this act is still honored and used to bring joy to the daily lives of others. In addition to feeding their own families and friends and hosting guests, it's common for individuals and companies to create incentives to feed others on a large scale. If you travel to any Muslim country in the Mediterranean during Ramadan, you'll find large tables set up in alleys where meals are served to fasting people for free on a nightly basis for the entire month.

The feast of Saint Anthony of Padua is a festival that still inspires communality in Italy. During the 13th century, a young woman left her baby alone, and he drowned. When she returned and found that he wasn't breathing, she prayed to Saint Anthony, offering to donate a quantity of bread equal to the weight of her son if he brought him back to life. And he did. From that moment on began the tradition of parents giving bread to protect their children. Even today, in the church of Crotone, Italy, and other places, there is a ceremony for the blessing of the bread. For this reason, there are also many organizations that follow this tradition, such as the work of the Pane di Sant'Antonio movement, which provides bread and nutritious meals, as well as the worldwide organization Bread for the Poor.

These traditions of offering bread as a prayer began in Ancient Egypt during pagan times. Today, we may have different beliefs, but I still believe in the power of bread, of hope itself, and in the sense of community that these traditions inspire.

In a more urgent sense of care being needed, Greek islanders from Lesvos were recently nominated for the Nobel Prize for their acts in feeding and caring for thousands of refugees arriving on their tiny island. It wasn't their physical duty or responsibility, but many of the islanders felt a strong sense of *filoxenía* (*xenia* means the law or custom of offering protection and hospitality to strangers and is the opposite of xenophobia). The notion of hospitality is so fundamental to human civilized life that its patron was Zeus Xenios, the god who protected strangers.

Research has shown that self-esteem, mood, and compassion can all be greatly improved by doing acts of kindness for others. Doing good things for others decreases blood pressure and *cortisol* (the stress hormone). These are just a few examples, but they show how community-based initiatives can have a direct and meaningful impact on our lives, society, and well-being. Finding pleasurable ways to give back to yourself and your community creates a win-win situation for everyone involved.

CULINARY METAPHORS FOR LIFE

"You are what you eat."

"The greater the food the greater the affection."

"At the table no one ages."

"The food you like is better digested."

These are just a few of the countless metaphors about food used daily in the Mediterranean region. Whether they're said in Arabic, French, Greek, Hebrew, Italian, Spanish, or Turkish, you'll likely hear these phrases while visiting a Mediterranean country. From a boarder perspective, people don't just say these statements, they live them. Dissecting each and every metaphor provides valuable lessons that can enhance our daily lives.

One of the most well-known aphorisms of French professor Jean Anthelme Brillat-Savarin, who wrote *The Physiology of Taste* (Vintage) and whose works offered a great deal to the science of *gastronomy* (the science of good eating), is "Tell me what you eat, and I shall tell you what you are." In other words, the better the food (in terms of quality and freshness), the better the person. The Mediterranean approach to food is that you should eat the best of what you can afford and offer the best food possible to yourself, your family, and your guests. Eating well is not seen as frivolous, nor does it mean you're a foodie or someone who is obsessed with the pleasures of the palate; it's a human right and responsibility.

You often hear Americans say about various Mediterranean cultures that people there tend to "take food very seriously." This is because people realize the important implications of food on physical, spiritual, and psychological well-being. In addition, they recognize food and the pleasures of dining as being something that everyone can partake in. Because we need food to survive anyway, we might as well make the most out of each and every meal, as well as every morsel that we put in our mouths and what we drink as well.

"The food is equal to the affection" is a traditional Arabic expression. I've seen this type of mentality play out in my own Southern Italian roots, as well as in Greek, Israeli, Spanish, and Turkish homes. There is an overwhelming notion that the better you feed someone, the more you care for them. It's so commonplace to be treated this way that if I'm ever in a situation where I'm not welcomed with an abundance of great food, I wonder whether the host or hostess cares about me at all! Sometimes, after serving what would be a very generous and lovely meal by American standards, I've been pulled aside and apologized to in private. Once, for example, my relatives in Italy served my business partner and me an ample seafood-based meal complete with several appetizers, a fish course with multiple types of seafood and side dishes, salad, fruit and nuts, and dessert. Even though I could never have dreamt of finishing the food that was there, I also realized that the hostess normally serves a lot more, and I began feeling a bit insecure. The next day, she apologetically pulled me aside and explained that she had created such a simple meal because the day before she had a procedure done on her knee and it bothered her to stand on her feet.

I tell that story time and time again because it perfectly exemplifies the type of care that people place on feeding one another. Our hostess could've easily ordered food from a restaurant, or told us to fend for ourselves (a knee procedure is certainly a good reason for not being able to cook!), but she wanted to create something for us with her own hands and preferred to show her care with a pared-down meal than to give us something made by someone else. Because I don't get to spend that much time there, she wanted to give me the gift of her own home cooking, to make as much as she possibly could to show her care, and to ensure that the meal was healthful and delicious.

That example is extreme, and there is no need for people to go to those lengths to be healthful and enjoy the Mediterranean lifestyle. But, I believe it's a beautiful goal to strive toward to ensure that the food you serve and eat exemplifies your affections in the best way possible.

"At the table no one ages" is an expression that is said and felt at Italian meals, as well as at typically lengthy meals in other places in the Mediterranean. There, people usually indulge in one very long meal per day. Typically it's lunch, but sometimes, depending upon people's schedules or whether it's a Sunday or a holiday, it may be dinner instead. The tradition of sitting around the table and slowly eating various courses or types of healthful foods with loved ones is the gold standard for daily infusions of well-being.

Psychologically, this tradition is rewarding because people's minds are calm at the table. At a very basic human level, eating and the awareness that food is available and abundant is calming to the psyche. The additional benefit of having people you care for around you helps to relieve stress. Longer dining times mean better digestion, and a wide variety of foods offer more nutrition. Camaraderie while dining helps you to absorb more nutrients from the food and actually eat less, even though there is more around to choose from.

"The food enjoyed is better digested" is another popular saying. This phrase underscores the importance of eating food that's pleasurable. Of course, if that food is already intrinsically healthful to begin with, the takeaways are even greater. I've never heard about anyone discussing "cheat days" while dieting or working out in Italy. Unless

(continued)

(continued)

they're on a very severe diet for a specific reason, most people in the Mediterranean region intersperse the foods they enjoy the most with a strong foundation of what's already nutritionally sound.

Muslims in the North African and Levantine portions of the Mediterranean are especially careful to feed babies, the sick, and the elderly the foods they enjoy most. There is a *hadith* (a saying or teaching of the Prophet Mohammed) that actually recommends feeding the ill foods they most enjoy. There are many examples that explain how the Prophet's wife, Aisha, would make him a dish called *tharid*, with lamb stock and toasted bread, which would help to nurse him back to good health. Whether it's chicken soup, tharid, or just a favorite food, a taste of something you really love when you aren't feeling your best can give you the extra incentive you need to heal.

Food is philosophy and feeling

Eating what you like and what's good for you is only the beginning of the equation for people in the Mediterranean region. People eat certain foods in order to:

» **Promote their culinary traditions.** Many traditional recipes in the Mediterranean region are at risk of falling out of fashion. Certain pasta shapes in Italy, breads in Greece, and sesame candies in Morocco, for example, are made only by a few people. As a result, people in these countries make a conscious effort to eat more of these foods so they don't become forgotten, especially when they speak to their own culture's traditions.

» **Show support for artisan producers.** The formation of co-ops to promote local and sustainable food and drinks across the Mediterranean is on the rise. Many residents choose to pay higher prices from producers they know in order to promote high-quality and artisan products in their own communities.

» **Make a statement.** Many people in the Mediterranean region eat a certain way or adapt a certain philosophy about food based upon the teachings of a particular philosopher, teacher, or historical figure. Each time they decide what to eat, they reason as if they *were* that person. This approach is a very common approach, and it makes people feel as if their eating has a specific role to play in a particular philosophy.

» **Pass down knowledge.** Eating styles are a way for people to show their commitment to passing down cultural attitudes and particular recipes or traditions from one generation to the next.

» **Heal their bodies.** Choosing certain foods that heal or prevent specific illnesses is a common way for people to eat in the Mediterranean region.

>> **Follow spiritual guidelines.** Whether you're in the North African or Eastern portion of the Mediterranean, many people eat a certain way in accordance with their religious beliefs. Fasting of the three monotheistic faiths (Christianity, Judaism, and Islam), as well as kosher and halal dietary guidelines, play an important role in daily diets and what's commonly eaten on various days. In Rome, for example, it's still common to serve fish on Fridays. Originally, Roman Catholics ate seafood on Fridays and didn't eat meat all weekend long until after taking the Eucharist at Mass on Sundays. Although most Romans no longer get weekly Communion at church, the tradition of serving fish at trattorias in the Eternal City is still common.

CONTEMPLATING THE COSMOS

We tend to think about food in terms of nutrients. The spiritual food that you feed your mind and body is also essential to your health. Many people never stop to think about spiritual food, but I find that the more of it you get, the less hungry you'll be, and the less you'll need to rely on food alone to "fill" you.

As a professional chef and writer, for example, I began to notice that I would always get hungry at certain times while I was sitting at my desk and writing. When I was cooking for long hours in the kitchen, though, I wouldn't get hungry at all. It sounds absurd to think that you could be completely engaged in preparing large amounts of food and be surrounded by it, yet not be hungry. There is scientific research, however, that illustrates how our bodies benefit from being around the aroma of food. We're genetically designed to feel comforted hormonally when we smell food being prepared. Our bodies are sent a signal that sustenance is on its way, and we aren't at risk of starving.

When we're sitting at a desk or in an area with no food or aromas of it, however, our bodies go into panic mode and our stress response is activated because, at a very basic level, our cells think we're at a risk for starvation. For this reason, many people working in offices feel hungry and may even eat more than people working in kitchens, despite the difference in physical activity of the two types of jobs.

My takeaway from learning this is that, in addition to taste, our senses of smell, touch, sight, and sound all help to "fill" us. In the Mediterranean region, you don't have to go far in order to smell the scent of fresh bread or something being simmered on the stove. Sumptuous fabrics or natural textures are usually available for the taking. Naturally pleasing sights abound, and music — whether it comes from the wild, a live musician, or a song streaming from the Internet — also provides great satisfaction. Surround yourself with as many sensory delights as possible before even tasting food.

(continued)

(continued)

That way, you'll eat less and absorb more nutrients while enjoying yourself in the process.

In order for our bodies to perform at their best, our minds need time to reflect upon not only our own emotions, but things larger than us as well. My good friend and colleague, Dr. Sam Pappas, always mentions the health benefits of the Ancient Greek practice of "contemplating the cosmos." The act of taking time each day, unplugged and uninterrupted, in our modern world can have a wonderful effect on our health.

Whether you're stargazing and contemplating the solar system, thinking about your role in society, or just taking time out to detach from the stresses of the day, turning your thoughts to something so large and immense can be very beneficial. Ancient philosophers used this technique. Different forms of *cosmology* (the study of the nature of the universe), whether they be physical, religious, or philosophical, are studied and practiced in the region. Different cultures and different people within those cultures have their own views, but contemplating your reason for existing, and finding a meaningful answer to that question, is linked to good health.

Those who have specific religious ideologies or philosophical beliefs often find comfort and sense out of contemplating and believing in the type of energy that exists beyond the physical universe. Adopting or following a belief system that answers our deepest questions while providing hope, structure, and reasons for our existence can provide a positive foundation upon which to build a healthy lifestyle. In the Mediterranean region, everything from mythology to ancient philosophy to monotheistic faiths, Buddhist beliefs, and New Age schools of thought can be called upon to make sense out of the uncontrollable aspects of our daily lives.

Believing that there is a higher order to the process of life is very empowering to many people in the region. The areas of the Mediterranean that are known for having people live the longest have experienced large amounts of adversity — wars and bombardments, famines, and natural disasters are no strangers to these places. At the same time, a sense of faith in the universe, our purpose, and creation itself has been one of the factors that has helped them to thrive. Regardless of which philosophy you adhere to, the mere act of deciding upon a particular way of thought and deriving emotional benefits from it set you up for mental and physical success.

Chapter **3**

Looking Forward to a Long and Healthful Life

In this chapter, I explain all the ways in which the Mediterranean lifestyle can improve your life and help you live longer and healthier. I introduce you to the scientific research that reveals why people can live better and longer by following a Mediterranean lifestyle. If you're looking for a little inspiration to fuel your lifestyle changes, this chapter is for you!

Seeing the Difference the Mediterranean Lifestyle Makes

In the Mediterranean region, many people believe that if you have a healthy mind, you'll have a healthy body. Many of the foods high in omega-3 fatty acids and citrus fruits eaten in a traditional Mediterranean diet play a role in overall cognitive function. But diet is only one of the lifestyle factors that improve mental performance. Increased social engagement, physical activity, sleep quality, daily activities, and other lifestyle factors help people to keep depression at bay and enjoy increased cognitive function, which in turn has a positive effect on the body.

REMEMBER

Diet alone can't guarantee overall optimal health. Lifestyle is a key component in well-being. The traditional Mediterranean lifestyle is known for enabling the people who practice it to live into the triple digits with relatively little illness. People who follow a Mediterranean lifestyle are increasing their likelihood of being able to live enjoyable and productive lives for a very long time.

Since the 1970s, more and more research has been done on the success rate of the Mediterranean diet. In recent decades, Mediterranean diet meal plans, recipes, and strategies have become much more widely available. Fortunately, today, people who have never stepped foot in the Mediterranean region are able to reap some of the rewards of the same healthful lifestyle.

If you only change your diet and you don't incorporate some of the other key lifestyle factors, you probably won't see the impressive and lasting results that are possible by adopting a Mediterranean lifestyle. I describe some of these results in the following sections.

Improving your health and preventing disease

In the United States and other places outside the Mediterranean region, disease such as obesity, heart disease, high blood pressure, high cholesterol, diabetes, or an autoimmune disease are often what lead people to the Mediterranean diet. In fact, more and more doctors are "prescribing" the Mediterranean diet to their patients. So, without even trying, the Mediterranean diet has become prescribed culinary medicine for many American patients.

What happens in these instances is that people who are already struggling with an illness are told that they should follow a Mediterranean diet. Sometimes, they're given a book or a pamphlet that outlines some healthful foods and good practices to follow. And that's a great place to start! Evidence shows that the anti-inflammatory and antioxidant benefits of following a Mediterranean diet can be effective in preventing and reversing many medical conditions when properly followed.

REMEMBER

The Mediterranean diet was used to *treat* illnesses since the days of Hippocrates. But when it is used as preventive "medicine," you can prevent many diseases, such as diabetes or heart disease, from occurring in the first place. The good news is that one of the reasons the diet is so popular and commonly "prescribed" by doctors is that it has an extremely high compliance rate. The Mediterranean way of eating deems no food completely "off limits," is easy to follow, offers endless recipes for delicious dishes to choose from, and has many health payoffs, even in the beginning.

By increasing physical activity, getting better-quality sleep, socializing, and engaging in meaningful regular activities, in addition to getting the proper nutrition, diseases can not only be treated but prevented. This is the goal of the Mediterranean lifestyle: to keep illness away to begin with.

Following a Mediterranean lifestyle has been known to:

>> Reduce the chances of developing heart disease by 47 percent.

>> Reduce incidence and symptoms of Parkinson's and Alzheimer's diseases.

>> Increase longevity.

>> Increase good gut bacteria, known as the *gastrointestinal microbiome.*

>> Prevent cancer and tumor growth.

>> Reduce the risk of death from heart disease and cancer.

>> Prevent and reverse diabetes, hypertension, attention deficit hyperactivity disorder (ADHD), and obesity.

Whether you want to reverse an illness that you're already dealing with, or prevent yourself and your loved ones from getting sick, incorporating as many aspects of the Mediterranean lifestyle into your daily life as possible will produce results. A Mediterranean diet combined with physical activity, good amounts of sleep, and daily functionality will help you to achieve your mental and physical health goals.

Living longer and better

What you have to gain by following the Mediterranean lifestyle includes better overall health and increased, better-quality performance. As a society, following a Mediterranean lifestyle will reduce healthcare costs. As an individual, you'll save money by staying healthy and avoiding large medical bills in the future. And for families, in addition to staying away from illness and saving on healthcare, many of the daily activities promoted in the Mediterranean lifestyle are fun, inexpensive ways to pass down traditions to future generations.

So many people automatically associate the idea of aging with getting sick. The thought of living longer when you aren't feeling well and not enjoying life to its fullest isn't very appealing. But it doesn't have to be that way! What's attractive about the Mediterranean lifestyle is that it allows people to enjoy themselves well into the latter parts of their lives and be more productive and active much later in life as well.

Often in the Mediterranean, you'll see senior citizens deftly making their way up a hilly path, walking briskly by on stairs, and staying up into the wee hours playing instruments or cards with friends. This is the way I would like to envision *my* golden years.

Worldwide acceleration of aging is set to become one of the 21st century's most significant social transformations. By 2050, the number of people over 60 years old is supposed to double, and by 2100 the number is expected to triple! A more promising and proactive look at aging is needed not only on an individual basis, but on a global one as well.

What the Experts Have to Say

Diet is just one healthful aspect of the Mediterranean lifestyle, but it certainly has been getting its fair share of attention in the American media these days! *U.S. News & World Report* named it the best diet in several categories for several years in a row. But that comes as no surprise to the people in the Mediterranean region who have been following it their entire lives.

The combination of a lifetime of enjoyable meals that taste great and just happen to be good for you is almost too good to be true! One of the most attractive attributes of the diet is that it doesn't ask you to give up anything or deprive yourself. It's a simple strategy that requires exercise, consuming the majority of calories from foods that are good for you, and reserving those that aren't for special occasions.

The following sections walk through what historical and modern research has to say about the Mediterranean way of life.

WHAT DOCTORS HAVE TO SAY

More and more medical doctors in England and the United States are "prescribing" the Mediterranean lifestyle to their patients to achieve optimal health. According to Dr. Sam Pappas (https://pappashealth.com), an award-winning physician certified in internal medicine who specializes in optimal wellness through a Mediterranean lifestyle:

> The Mediterranean diet and lifestyle have their origins in the culture and habits of the historically vibrant and consequential Greek island of Crete. Crete's unique location allowed its inhabitants to absorb, create, and share its health and diet

knowledge with the known *oikos* [an Ancient Greek word referring to home or household] of the Hellenic community and later the Greco-Roman world. These Greeks and their Mediterranean forebears demonstrated strength and resiliency in the physics and metaphysics of survival and flourishing through this unique diet and lifestyle that has remained virtually unchanged over millennia. This diverse diet is full of wholesome and satisfying foods and drinks made of bioprotective nutrients, coupled with a culture that emphasizes movement and the unity of family and village, and is placed in a physically healing environment of warmth and the sea. All of this leads anyone partaking in such a Mediterranean diet and lifestyle to achieve optimal health, prevent diseases, reduce stress, and improve quality of life.

Dr. Simon Poole, a medical doctor in Cambridge, England, has been recommending evidence-based Mediterranean nutrition for his patients for many years, seeing real differences in their physical and mental health as they learn more about delicious foods that confer significant benefits. Now involved in teaching, international speaking, and writing on the subject, Dr. Poole is renowned for his passionate advocacy for communicating the science of the diet to the public in a way that can promote a healthy, sustainable, and enjoyable way of life.

Dr. John Rosa, owner and supervisor of Accessible Beltway Clinics (which is composed of 17 clinics in Maryland and Virginia), author, and White House consultant across Republican and Democratic administrations, has this to say about the Mediterranean diet and lifestyle:

> The Mediterranean way of life is a most fortunate one. The land and sea are blessed with an abundance of great vegetation, fish, and shellfish. The climate is exceptional, which results in more time spent enjoying the outdoors. The door to great health has several locks, and the Mediterranean lifestyle holds all the keys. The sun boosts your immune system by producing vitamin D while you tend to your garden. Food is most nutritious when prepared at home with home ingredients. The act of saying grace is, in itself, a digestive aid because it makes us present and appreciative of God's abundance. The table is not just filled with food but people. The community meal of family and/or friends is therapeutic on a mental health scale of the highest level. This is followed by a walk and that simple shot of black coffee. Finally, early to bed and early to rise [are in] keeping with the millions of years of evolutionary sleep patterns according to daylight. Family, friends, food, faith, and fun. Yup, it's that easy!

Historical studies on the Mediterranean lifestyle

One study that experts everywhere turn to when discussing the Mediterranean diet and lifestyle is the Seven Countries Study (www.sevencountriesstudy.com), which was the first large-scale study that inspired an American and Western interest in the benefits of eating and living the way people in pre–World War II Mediterranean countries (namely, Italy, Spain, and Greece) did.

These studies, made famous by Dr. Ancel Keys (1904–2004), were pioneering in that they demonstrated how serum cholesterol, blood pressure, diabetes, and smoking are universal risk factors for coronary artery disease. Dr. Keys was a University of Minnesota researcher who demonstrated how the apparent epidemic of heart attacks in middle-aged American men was related to their lifestyle and possibly modifiable physical characteristics.

Revolutionary for their time, Dr. Keys' findings proved that people could take control of their health and their lives by taking cues from the Mediterranean region. His work paved the way for Mediterranean diet and lifestyle advocates to adopt this approach in their medical practices, books, consultancies, and classes.

Modern research

TIP

This section gets into the weeds on some modern research into Mediterranean lifestyle, but if you're not interested in reading about the science, here are some simple facts to keep in mind:

» Despite being difficult to research, it has been proven to improve both mental and physical health significantly.

» Following a Mediterranean lifestyle can significantly reduce your risk of a wide-range of diseases.

» Adherence to a Mediterranean lifestyle increases longevity.

» Doctors, nutritionists, dietitians, and other medical professionals in the United States and abroad recommend the Mediterranean lifestyle.

REMEMBER

Diet is an important *element* in lifestyle, but it's not the whole story. Physical exercise and diet *combined* are the most important lifestyle factors to losing weight. The additional lifestyle factors of socializing and engaging in community activities, getting a good night's sleep and napping, having a positive outlook, engaging in pleasurable activities, developing effective strategies for dealing with adversity, and practicing relaxation techniques are additional factors leading to optimal well-being.

TECHNICAL STUFF

Now, for some of the science:

» Currently neurodegenerative diseases are becoming more and more prevalent. In 2010, 35.6 million people were reported to have suffered from dementia, and that number is expected to nearly double every two decades.

In 2018, MDPI published an article entitled "Mediterranean Lifestyle in Relation to Cognitive Health: Results from the HELIAD Study" (www.mdpi.com/2072-6643/10/10/1557), which concluded that four lifestyle factors, "namely diet, physical activity, sleep, and functionality" had a beneficial influence on the elderly.

» In the Hellenic Longitudinal Investigation of Ageing and Diet (HELIAD) study (https://pubmed.ncbi.nlm.nih.gov/24993387), 1,716 patients who were over 65 years of age participated. Because nonclinical cognitive impairment has been associated with increased mortality rates and other conditions, analyzing the risk of this phenomenon was essential. At the end of the study, worse lifestyle was observed in dementia patients and better Total Lifestyle Index (TLI), an overall lifestyle pattern for people living in the Mediterranean including diet, physical activity, sleep and daily living activities with social/intellectual aspects, was associated with better global cognitive functioning. Better diet was related to better memory and visual-spatial and language function in the same study.

» A Spanish study at the Universidad de Navarra (https://journals.sagepub.com/doi/full/10.1177/2167702616638651) analyzed the correlation between the Mediterranean lifestyle in addition to diet and the risk of depression. The 8½-year study of 11,800 people found that those who adhered to a Mediterranean lifestyle reduced their risk of depression by 50 percent.

» In 2015–2016, a manuscript published by the U.S. National Library of Medicine at the National Institutes of Health (www.ncbi.nlm.nih.gov/pmc/articles/PMC5902736) reviewed the recent relevant evidence of the effects of the Mediterranean diet and lifestyle on health. They were found to represent the "gold standard in preventive medicine, probably due to the harmonic combination of many elements with antioxidant and anti-inflammatory properties, which overwhelm any single nutrient or food item." Their findings included 19 new reports that showed that the Mediterranean diet and lifestyle reduced the risk of heart attack, stroke, mortality, heart failure, and disability, as well as preventing cognitive decline and breast cancer.

ANCIENT INSPIRATION FOR MODERN TIMES

By looking to the past for inspiration, we can clearly see how our ancient ancestors used the tenets of the Mediterranean lifestyle to improve their quality of life, heal themselves, and ward off illnesses. Sometimes people are intimidated by delving into the Mediterranean lifestyle because there is no specific set of rules to follow the way there

(continued)

(continued)

are in many modern diets. But it's the freedom associated with the Mediterranean lifestyle that makes it so appealing and has enabled it to stand the test of time!

Over the years, many of my students and readers have asked me to create specific meal plans and schedules that they must follow in order to adhere to this rich and rewarding lifestyle. I've always been honored by their requests, and flattered that they would follow exactly what I would tell them to do, but I've always resisted the temptation to give them a set of rules. Why? Because, at its core, the Mediterranean lifestyle works because there is no one set of rules that works for every single person.

Different people, at different ages, and in different periods of their life have different mental, emotional, and physical needs. It would be a huge disservice to the world to unveil a blanket plan for everyone.

In the sixth century BCE, the revolutionary Greek mathematician and philosopher Pythagoras chose to call my ancestral hometown of Crotone (then called Kroton), Italy, home. There he set up the most important school in ancient Magna Grecia, where he taught math, nutrition, poetry, and music. Pythagoras himself was a devout vegetarian. He's also known as the "Father of Vegetarianism" in the West. He believed that human beings could reincarnate as animals, so he avoided eating living things and demanded that his students, followers, and disciples do the same.

Pythagoras had such an aversion to eating meat that he even forbade his followers from eating fava beans because he felt that their constitution was similar to that of living beings. Despite his personal feelings, however, when he advised his son-in-law, Milo, an ancient wrestler and Olympic champion and one of the greatest athletes of all time, on his diet, he suggested that Milo eat meat, because the intense physical strength of his profession required him to do so.

This very early act of individualism was profound, and it has been a lesson for all proponents of the Mediterranean lifestyle to follow for millennia. Pythagoras's diet and logic was followed by future philosophers such as Hippocrates and Epicurus. His dietary teachings became known as the Greek diet, and centuries later that became known as the Mediterranean diet.

The Mediterranean diet that we promote today is based largely upon the Greek diet and the traditional foodways of ancient Crete. Subsequent studies and research from places like Sardinia, Italy, and Ikaria, Greece, help to illustrate that the lifestyle is alive and well in many places in the Mediterranean. Even locations such as Morocco, Egypt, and Israel, which don't automatically pop up in people's minds as being beacons of the Mediterranean lifestyle, offer shining examples of how we can extract delicious and pleasurable techniques to enjoy a long, healthful, enjoyable, and meaningful life.

Chapter **4**

Achieving the Mediterranean Lifestyle Abroad

When I talk with people in the United States about following a Mediterranean lifestyle, I often hear, "It's easy to do if you live on a remote island or somewhere in the South of France, but I have a really busy life, and I just can't live that way here." Yes, living in a place where this style of life is the norm may make it easier to follow, but there's no reason why you can't achieve similar results wherever you live.

In this chapter, I explain how to live your best life by making the Mediterranean lifestyle work for you, no matter where you currently reside.

Lifestyle Habits to Enjoy as Often as Possible

Even though no one ever talks about it, I sometimes think that people living outside the Mediterranean have an advantage when it comes to incorporating various aspects of the traditional lifestyle into their daily activities. Why? Because when you've grown up in a place, you may take it for granted.

Many young people in the Mediterranean region don't appreciate their customs and long to go abroad to live in cities and appreciate other ways of life. The often free daily luxuries that they experience are easy to take for granted until you see other places in the world, where modern lifestyles have robbed people of those daily pleasures.

Luckily, it's never too late to get our health, time, and lives back under our own control. Even people in the region are experiencing rapid rates of modernization, which requires constantly adjusting their schedules, habits and customs in order to lead healthy lives. With the easy-to-incorporate, inexpensive, and pleasurable tips in this section, making the most of your situation is a cinch.

TIP

When incorporating the habits in this section, I recommend keeping a journal. Incorporate a new item each day or week, depending upon how much time and energy you want to dedicate to it. Before bed, take time to write down any of your efforts in this area and if you noticed any synergies or positive feedback. It won't take long before you witness inspiration to continue.

Practicing gratitude

The Mediterranean region is certainly not the first or only region in which people have benefitted from actively expressing gratitude and giving thanks as a means of leading a better life. That said, I'm always pleased to continue to witness and learn about new ways to practice gratitude in my own life, and the Mediterranean region never fails to deliver inspiration.

Here are the most commonly practiced forms of gratitude in the region:

>> Giving thanks for the small things

>> Being grateful for larger accomplishments, blessings, and life events

>> Using gratitude to override a negative situation

>> Expressing gratitude toward others and past events

TECHNICAL STUFF

The word *gratitude* is derived from the Latin word *gratia,* which means grace or gratefulness. The meaning of the word is to experience a thankful appreciation for receiving something. Positive psychology explains that, because this process involves recognizing that what you're thankful for came from a source outside ourselves, feeling gratitude enables you to connect to others and the world at large more effectively. Research shows that gratitude leads to greater happiness through positive emotions, which in turn improve our health, help us to cope with difficult situations, and enhance our interpersonal relations.

Giving thanks for the small things is a quick and easy way to feel better instantly. Because the "small" things that we're fortunate to have every day — water, fresh air, the ability to breathe, a loved one — are things we can't do without, it makes sense that we give thanks for them, even though, often times, we don't have to do anything to enjoy them. The act of gratitude helps us to feel happier, connect with the outside world, and affirm our place in the universe.

Being grateful for larger accomplishments easy to do in modern culture. We're used to hearing people giving thanks for things they've wanted for a long time — a new job, a baby, a new car or home, a promotion, an award, and so on. In addition to personally feeling thankful, or giving thanks to a higher power for these milestones, most people in the Mediterranean would do something to be able to share their accomplishments with the community — through a public act of charity, a large celebration, smaller gifts for others, or social media posts — in order to demonstrate their gratitude outwardly.

Because these opportunities don't usually happen on a daily basis, it's important to give thanks for the things you tend to take for granted as well. When people in the Mediterranean region hear about one of their friends or family members achieving one of these important events, they often buy them a gift, invite them to celebrate, or at least treat them to a coffee or tea, especially if they aren't involved in the actual celebration itself.

Using gratitude to override a negative situation was something I was unfamiliar with until I began to spend time in Muslim countries in the Mediterranean region, where it's common to hear *alhumdullilah* (thank God) at even the most trying of times. The first time I witnessed this was when someone was talking about a loved one who had just been in a car accident. I was shocked. "Who would be able to give thanks at a moment like that?" I wondered to myself, filled with pity for the suffering relative.

With time, I witnessed situations like that over and over again, and you can see it for yourself on Arabic language news programs or in popular movies and TV shows. One day, when I had learned a little bit more about energy and the law of attraction, I realized that by thanking God in a horrible circumstance, we can immediately call upon help. It shifts the negative out of the situation and allows the possibility of a solution, or at bare minimum some kind of comfort. It also acknowledges a higher power who can rectify the situation, and the fact that things could always be worse than they are.

Like all ancient cultures, the cultures in the Mediterranean aren't strangers to difficult times. Research has shown that praying in the most disastrous of times can lead to not only relief, but also to what many people consider to be miracles as well.

Expressing gratitude toward others and for past events is something that people in the Mediterranean spend a lot of time doing. This is one of the most common forms of "table talk" no matter where you are. Expressing gratitude toward others helps both parties enjoy positive emotions, and the person who is being thanked will have a happy emotional response knowing that they or their action is appreciated. In Italy, expressing gratitude for past events could be a national pastime. Italians love to reminisce, and to give thanks at the same time is especially rewarding. Many artistic creations — paintings, poems, songs, recipes — are made with gratitude for something or someone in mind.

TIP

Here are four easy ways to give more thanks:

>> **Start small.** Imagine your life without the daily essentials you take for granted and give thanks for each of them, starting with air and water.

>> **Write down a list of large accomplishments that you've achieved in the last year, the last five years, and throughout your life.** Give a heartfelt thanks for each of them.

>> **Look at some past seemingly negative situations in your life with a new outlook.** How could that event have held hidden blessings? Write down your findings.

>> **Write a list of ten people who have done amazing things for you — either in the past day, the past year, or your life.** Spend time writing a deep letter explaining how their actions made you feel and how much you appreciate them. If the person is no longer in your life, thank them mentally and put the letter away. If they are still in your life, perfect the letter, and send it to them or give it to them in person.

These simple and effective techniques can be used to feel better anytime. In the Mediterranean region, they're especially effective because the cultures at large believe in them. That means that if someone needs encouragement or cheering up, they can count on their friends and family to remind them of what they have to be grateful for. I'm fortunate that I have created this type of network even in the United States, and my friends and I do this for each other. Just as having an accountability partner that you exercise with to keep your body in shape, a gratitude partner can help you stay on track emotionally.

Enjoying meals and physical activity with others

The Mediterranean Diet Pyramid (see Chapter 13) is what many doctors and nutritionists use to teach the tenets of this healthful eating pattern to people worldwide. The base of the pyramid shows the importance that Mediterranean cultures place on enjoying meals with others and being physically active. Regardless of religion, ethnicity, or language, the people of the Mediterranean region share a common desire to spend time eating and socializing with friends.

Whether it's a local proverb or a religious recommendation, no Mediterranean country is short on sayings that consistently remind people of the importance of eating together. In the Muslim countries of the Mediterranean region, there are even prophetic sayings encouraging believers to choose who they eat with before they decide what to eat, just as the Greek philosopher Epicurus did many centuries earlier.

Regardless of the particular culture in the region, people go out of their way to plan meals together, which has been linked to increased longevity, better digestion, and eating less. I love hearing stories from readers who maintain these traditions all over the world.

Even today, most people in the Mediterranean find it unpleasant to eat alone. Fortunately, in many places, work and school schedules revolve around mealtimes. When they don't, families change their schedules in order to be able to eat together — at least for one meal per day. If you haven't reaped the benefits of this lifestyle, I highly recommend seeking out family, friends, coworkers, and neighbors with whom you can enjoy meals more often.

Every country and culture around the Mediterranean has its own way of encouraging people to eat. Residents on the Mediterranean island of Sardinia, for example, are ten times more likely to live past the age of 100 than people in the United States. Researchers who studied this remarkable longevity found that daily *communal* (family-style) eating was commonplace, and they credited the overall well-being of residents to this tradition. The researchers concluded that there is something extremely satisfying and comforting about knowing that, no matter how difficult life gets, at lunchtime you'll be surrounded by loved ones. It adds a deep sense of psychological security, which, in turn, has a positive effect on health and happiness.

It's often difficult, given our demanding work schedules, to schedule time to spend with others, but the benefits are truly worth the effort. Even when it isn't possible to be with someone else (in my case when I'm writing at home and I'm alone), I send a message to a loved one and arrange to call them when I'm eating. It has become a "thing" with my family and writer friends — and it makes me feel great that I can catch up with others and my work at the same time.

Start planning shared meals and physical activities with others. When planning out your week, make sure you have a shared meal and a shared activity every day. The shared meal may need to be via Facetime, and the shared activity may need to be with a neighbor, a coworker, or someone you've just met through a meetup group designed for people with similar interests. The goal is to increase these activities and enjoy them more. Finding the mix that you like best may take time, but that's part of the fun! If you aren't already regularly eating or doing activities with others, enjoy the process of making this happen.

TIP

Here are some ways to enjoy communal activities more:

>> **Notice pockets in your day in which you could spend time with someone else.** It could be a pre-breakfast walk, lunch at the office, dinner outside, gardening, exercising, shopping, or running errands.

>> **Write down names of people you know who might find it fun to share those activities with you.** Then contact them and compare schedules. If you can't meet in person, you can meet virtually (via video calls)!

>> **Start with just one or two additional events each week, and gradually build up to daily events.**

If you already have a schedule full of meaningful times that you share with others, give thanks for that, knowing that it's giving you more health benefits than you can count.

Taking life and yourself lightly

One of the secrets to success in the Mediterranean region is not to take life or yourself too seriously. Taking things with a grain of salt has helped people over-come stressors — both large and small — throughout the entire area. Whether it's expressed through the noteworthy Egyptian sense of humor or the classic *dolce far niente* (the act of "sweet doing nothing"), which the Neapolitans have made an artform, there is a lot of regional motivation to let go of stress.

Some people explain this from a historical standpoint. Obviously, they say, if you're accustomed to living in an area where a volcano could erupt at any given moment, or one where war seems to break out overnight, the people who inhabit those places will most likely be adept at making the most out of every moment that they aren't in physical danger.

Others claim that millennia worth of philosophically rich doctrines and spiritual motivation have caused people in the Mediterranean to seize not only the day, but also every moment they can and not to worry too much about things that are out of their control. Personally, I believe there are also energetic components that help people in the region to take themselves less seriously.

When I'm walking in my ancestral hometown of Crotone, Calabria, down the streets of Rome, or in Old Cairo, just to name a few places, I always feel a sense of calm come over me. The streets may be busy and sounds may be coming from everywhere, but in those places, I feel safe and secure. This is because it both humbles and grounds me to think that the likes of Pythagoras, emperors, caliphs, and prophets walked those same streets. I begin to feel insignificant (in a healthy way) and to realize that my to-do list and the majority of the things I may be stressed over probably were not an issue a thousand years ago — and because of this, it's easier for me to let go.

Stress can increase cortisol levels and inflammation, and cause you to be less happy and healthy. But taking life less seriously can help you to calm down, relax, focus, and eliminate excess stress. In the beginning, it can be challenging to let go of things that you've held onto so tightly for long periods of time. Often, our self-worth and identity get tied up with our ultra-serious approach to certain topics.

TIP

Here are some Mediterranean-style questions to consider when you become upset:

>> Will this matter a hundred years from now?

>> Is what I'm worrying about or obsessing over worth negatively affecting my health?

>> Does this issue apply to me personally, and is it my responsibility, or am I just emotionally taking it on because the topic matters to me?

>> What can I do to feel better in this moment?

Asking yourself these simple questions, and being honest with yourself about the answers, can help you overcome unnecessary worry and take life more lightly. If you're obsessing over something because it's important to you, your strategy is actually faulty. You need a clear head and focus to resolve any issue, so it's better to take things more lightly so you'll be more effective in getting what you want.

Small Habits with Big Payoffs

The combination of healthful, homegrown (or as close to homegrown as possible) foods, along with pleasurable sounds and the communal/physical activity of dancing, provide people in the Mediterranean region with daily access to comfort and joy. The more of these things that you include in your daily life, the healthier and happier you'll be.

Eating as close to home as possible

In the Mediterranean region, eating close to home doesn't mean selecting a restaurant that's near your home or place of work, although it may. It typically refers to what are called *zero-kilometer foods* (foods that are grown less than 1 kilometer [a little more than ½ mile] from your home). Fortunately this trend is spreading!

There are many good reasons to want to eat foods grown close to your home. Nutritionally speaking, our bodies crave the nutrients in the foods that are in season in the areas where we live. For example, where I live, dandelions start to pop up in the springtime. Dandelion roots and leaves are known to have powerful detoxifying and antioxidant properties, which help our bodies transform into the warmer months ahead (in addition to many other benefits). My body doesn't require the same nutrients after fall when we head into winter, so it wouldn't make sense for me to eat them from elsewhere at that time. Instead, my body *does* need the nutrients from fall produce — apples, squash, and broccoli, for example — which I can also get in my area.

Whether you shop at a local farmer's market, belong to a community-supported agriculture (CSA) program, or grow things in your own garden, these are all steps in the right direction. Even buying produce grown in your area while it's in season from the grocery store is better than buying the bulk of your meal ingredients from other places. Adopting a "buy local" mentality and experimenting with growing your own foods will have a positive impact on the environment and give you a satisfying sense of supporting your community as well.

TIP

Here are some ways to enjoy more local foods:

>> Join a CSA or other program where local foods are delivered to you.

>> Start your own garden.

>> Use a windowsill, balcony, porch, or terrace to grow herbs and edible plants.

>> Shop at farmers markets and/or purchase more local produce from your supermarket.

With just a few small tweaks to your schedule, these activities will guarantee more flavor and nutrients. You can also really enjoy yourself in the process! Growing our own food gives a great sense of accomplishment and is especially fun for children. Supporting local farmers and businesses helps to improve community relations and commerce.

Music and dancing

Ah, the delights of music and dancing! Music is the quickest, fastest way to transport myself to the Mediterranean region, and I do it all day every day. I even enjoy music while I write and sleep. To me, life is too short to spend without being accompanied by beautiful sounds. Sometimes, reminiscent of the movie *Il Postino*, I record sounds when I'm in the Mediterranean region — the call to prayer in Morocco, sheep bleating in Egypt, the sea in Greece (or anywhere, really), the wind off the shore in Calabria, and the Grand Bazaar in Istanbul. When I get nostalgic for these places, I play the sounds.

Music has a very quick and direct effect on our moods, so playing what's appealing to you in any given moment is a wonderful way to feel good. In addition, it's great to play music that you enjoy from different countries while cooking and eating (bonus points if the music matches the cuisine). To most people in the Mediterranean region, regardless of the country, eating a meal without music is like watching a movie on mute — something is missing.

I often joke that our modern cultures have our priorities backward: We save music and dancing for special occasions, such as weddings or holidays, and then spend the rest of our days without them. Around the Mediterranean basin, however, each culture boasts a variety of traditional, classical, and modern styles of music and dance that are enjoyed as often as possible. It doesn't take much, for example, for people to break out into song and dance after a meal in Greece, Spain, Turkey, Egypt, and everywhere in between.

Many of the dances that are practiced in the Mediterranean region are done communally. In ancient times, the dances weren't just for fun; each one had a significance and related to the agricultural cycles, as well as important life events and rites of passages. Whether it's the *debka* danced in Lebanon, a Nubian folk dance in Egypt, one of the many Italian variations of the tarantella, or various Greek dances, performing them helps individuals and communities to connect, heal, and celebrate together. Dancing has helped each culture process and transform negative emotions, such as grief and sadness, while giving them joyous ways to commemorate happy ones as well.

In the case of the Greek dance called Zeibekiko, for example, it's a dance that's performed individually by a person — traditionally by a man, but now it's becoming popular with women as well — who has reached rock bottom and needs to dance in order to dance away the melancholy brought by someone who is away from their homeland. Also known as the eagle dance, Zeibekiko has no set moves, but rather allows the dancer to improvise their own emotions into meaning. It's believed that a true gentleman will only dance the Zeibekiko alone, so as to leave time and space for others to dance away their demons. Known as being a personal, transformational moment, Zeibekiko is not a celebratory, social dance, although it is gaining more attention as one nowadays. Originally, it was viewed as a highly personal, introspective moment that must be respected.

The Gnawa musicians of Morocco play a style of music with a ubiquitous sound that is said to represent the sounds that the chains and shackles placed on enslaved people made when they would dance. It's said to have special healing properties, and modern families have been known to pay Gnawa performers, which are extremely popular with tourists, to come to their homes and play for people who are suffering from all kinds of ailments — ranging from headaches to life-threatening diseases.

I had seen and heard Gnawa music live several times in Morocco, but it wasn't until I learned its history that it really made me realize the power of the human mind and spirit to be happy. It took me months to wrap my mind around the concept of enslaved people dancing to begin with. Many of us struggle to find reasons to be happy given the challenges of our daily lives. But those struggles pale in comparison to what it would be like to be enslaved. Hearing their story and speaking with the musicians really inspired me. It made me realize how much we take for granted. And it reminded me that we should use any excuse possible to dance and be happy.

I even started drawing parallels between the different types of music and dance styles in the Mediterranean region's history. This helped me come to the conclusion that we don't need a once-in-a-lifetime milestone to dance. In the Mediterranean, the desire to feel better is reason enough to dance, and when you start, you'll always be encouraged to continue. What's more, dancing can be a transporting therapy that may just help you edge your way up the emotional scale from even dark despair to contentment, happiness, and joy.

People in the United States and Europe are surprised to learn that belly dancing, for example, which many Westerners associate with seduction, actually involves specific movements that help women's overall health. It has been used since the beginning of time as a way for women to express themselves and their emotions. In addition to being practiced at celebrations (when it's thought to bring good luck), belly dancing is done by women at home to help re-integrate their bodies after giving birth and throughout various stages in life.

TIP

To add more Mediterranean-style joy to your life:

>> Surround yourself with the sounds and music that feels best to you.

>> Use cooking, exercise, or other daily activity as an excuse to listen to more music.

>> Dance as often as possible, whether you feel good or bad.

>> Discover new ways to incorporate more music and dance into your life — and don't save them for special occasions.

TECHNICAL STUFF

Did you know that music is so powerful that many vineyard owners in Italy play it on loudspeakers in their grape orchards so that the grapes will grow better and be more resistant to disease? Imagine what listening to pleasurable music can do to our bodies. It has been shown to reduce anxiety, blood pressure, and pain. It can also improve our cognitive function and sleep quality. This is because many emotions stem from our brains, in addition to our hearts. Certain types of music can cause our emotions to peak and increase the amount of a neurotransmitter called *dopamine,* which controls the brain's reward and pleasure centers. In addition to the physical benefits, dancing helps to reduce stress and increases levels of the feel-good hormone *serotonin,* which is reason alone to start doing it more often.

Water, steam, and relaxation

The relaxation that access to warm water provides is invaluable in terms of wellness. Turkish baths, thermal springs, saunas, and water itself are valued and prized in the Mediterranean region for their healing benefits. Most people, no matter their income bracket, culture, or lifestyle, incorporate one or more of these elements into their weekly rituals. I'm a huge proponent of all of them, but they're a little bit less commonplace in the United States, so we tend not to hear about them as much.

In the North African and Middle Eastern areas of the Mediterranean basin, *hamams* (Turkish baths) are usually stone and marble structures that have ample heated running water — an amazing luxury in the 10th century. In ancient times, the *medinas* (town centers) needed to have a public bath in order to be considered complete. These baths were always located next to the bread bakeries because the water was heated from the same oven.

Going to the bath used to be (and sometimes still is) a weekly ritual for many people. Originally, the baths were communal and separated by the sexes. In the baths, you could either wash yourself or pay someone else to wash you. The washing included an exfoliating scrub with a loofah, followed by soap, and oftentimes finished with essential oils. In addition to the intoxicating sensation of the steam, the aromas wafting from the baths are equally delicious.

The public baths remained a necessity until hot running water became commonplace in homes. Nowadays, however, they're still popular among both men and women in various forms. Many people, myself included, enjoy the spa versions, which you can experience in many urban centers across the Mediterranean region today, as well as in hotels and inns. Many people combine massages with their steam treatments and baths. Regardless, the combination of the hot steam, pleasant scents, and warm water have a profoundly relaxing effect on the body.

Saunas were also popular in antiquity. Many Asklepion-style temples and more modern healing centers in Greece and Turkey also promote this type of therapy. Asklepion became known as a healing complex located at the base of the Pergamon acropolis in Turkey. It was built in honor of Asclepius, the god of healing.

Asklepion was a term used in Ancient Greece to define a type of temple devoted to the god Asclepios, which acted as a healing center. Asklepios was the Ancient Greek god of healing, whose temples and healing sanctuaries were places the Greeks went to heal and recover — not just in Pergamon, but throughout the Greek and Roman Empire. Complete with saunas, baths, and gymnasiums, these centers offered services that are still appropriate to our healing today. Whether you have access to a sauna in your residence, gym, or local spa, paying a visit to one will offer relaxing and detoxifying benefits.

Your mind, body, and spirit will all benefit from a visit to the sauna. Regular trips to the sauna can help your body release heavy metals and toxins such as arsenic, cadmium, lead, and mercury. Known to promote relaxation, promote detoxification, and reduce blood pressure, studies also reveal that visiting the sauna four to seven times per week reduces the risk of death from cardiovascular disease by up to 58 percent.

Additional benefits of using a sauna include increased metabolism, weight loss, increased blood circulation, pain and inflammation reduction, antiaging benefits, skin and cell rejuvenation, improved cardiovascular function, improved immune function, and better sleep. Using the sauna is the perfect antidote to tired minds and muscles. But what if you don't have a sauna located near you, or what if it's difficult to get to one?

If you want to get the continuous benefits of a sauna at a fraction of the price, you can consider purchasing a home sauna. Starting at around $1,000, the prefabricated models offer many benefits. An even less expensive option is a portable sauna or sauna blankets that can cost between $200 to $500. These can be folded up, stored, and taken with you if a permanent version isn't an option.

In addition to steam, just plain old water has numerous benefits to our health. Along with drinking enough water and eating foods that contain large amounts of water (such as cucumbers, melon, and celery), watching and listening to water has very relaxing effects on the body.

Do you ever notice that being near water just seems to make people happy? It's not all in their heads. A great deal of research has proven that even proximity to water, hearing it, and envisioning it has benefits to our overall well-being. Whether you're near, in, on, or under clean water, the effects it can have on your system include lower stress and anxiety, an overall sense of well-being and happiness, and a lower heart and breathing rate.

Workouts in the water, such as water aerobics and swimming, are very safe and highly effective. Being near the water boosts creativity. In our daily lives and in literature and lore, you can see how it has been the perfect backdrop for romance and healing. Aquatic therapists use water as a medium to help treat and manage post-traumatic stress disorder (PTSD), addiction, anxiety disorders, autism, and more.

If you don't have frequent access to a beach, don't despair! You can get many great effects just by visiting a lake, pond, creek, river, or even a fountain. Listening to a recording of waves on the beach can help you relax before sleep and destress your days.

Want to relax more? Try incorporating these water-based rituals in your daily life:

>> Visit saunas and steam baths, or create your own as often as possible.

>> Listen to the sounds of the ocean, whether it is live or in a recording.

>> Visit sources of water — lakes, streams, oceans, rivers, and ponds — as often as possible.

>> Consider using a home sauna or sauna blanket.

Everyone responds differently to various stimuli — steam and water included — so be sure to add the elements into your life that are the easiest to incorporate and give you the most pleasure. The good news is, although this book offers many options, even a few small changes can bring large-scale results.

2

Making the Mediterranean Lifestyle Work for You

Chapter **5**

Making Meals a Priority

When we take the time to eat well, we're honoring not only nature but ourselves. Modern research has also proven that people who eat communally eat far more vegetables than those who eat alone and that they make better food choices when dining together. Contrary to popular belief, the more emphasis we place on regular mealtimes, quality food, and enjoying what we eat, the happier and healthier we'll be. The concept of communal dining is something that those living outside the Mediterranean region often struggle with, but this chapter offers inspirational ideas you can easily adopt.

Seeing Mealtimes as Sacred

If I had a magic wand that I could wave to make everyone successful on the Mediterranean diet, it would be one that makes them guard their mealtimes with the same fervor that they guard their most precious possessions. Eating the right foods and getting exercise alone won't provide as many lasting results and rewards that the Mediterranean lifestyle offers. In addition to nutrition, planned and pleasurable mealtimes set you up for psychological success. This, in turn, affects your hormone levels and metabolism. According to the Mental Health Foundation (www.mentalhealth.org.uk/a-to-z/d/diet-and-mental-health):

> Regular mealtimes . . . offer a sense of containment and familiarity and can evoke deep feelings of contentment and security. Humans need structure and routine. Mealtimes offer people the opportunity to stop, to stand still psychologically, to

reflect on their day and days ahead, and to listen to and interact with others. Mealtimes are also a grounding opportunity, a time when anxieties can be expressed and you can be listened to.

This "secret" is often the last thing on people's mind as they make the switch to a Mediterranean diet. This step seems hard because it's a seemingly big time commitment. It may also seem unattainable because much of the Western world has been taught to believe that time spent eating is time wasted, and that there are much better and more important, productivity-driven things that you can do with your time instead of spending it at the table. People are even doing away with tables in their homes in lieu of bars and islands where they can grab a quick bite or just sit in front of the TV as they binge-watch their favorite shows.

When you understand the import role that mental health and emotions play on your overall well-being and physical health, it becomes very easy to adopt legendary food writer M.F.K. Fisher's philosophy: "First we eat. Then we do everything else." Whether you consider yourself a "foodie" or not, the pleasures of the table and their health benefits far outweigh the inconvenience of starting a new habit. Having worked and lived throughout the Mediterranean region, I can honestly say that people in Southern Europe, North Africa, and all of the Levant share this mentality.

How this cultural tradition plays out in different countries is unique, but the end result is the same — the common belief that eating is one of life's greatest pleasures, one that we're fortunate enough to be able to take part in. For that reason, people organize their lives around their meals, and not the other way around. When in Italy, for example, almost everyone, whether you're in a business setting or a social setting, will start to get a little bit fidgety before 1 p.m. That's because they know that they need to be at home with their loved ones or outside with their friends, giving their bodies the nourishment and their minds the stability that they deserve and depend upon to function properly.

One of the major things that most people in the Mediterranean region have in their favor are work and school hours that allow long lunch leaves. Of course, this makes keeping mealtimes sacred much easier. I look forward to the day when people outside the Mediterranean can do the same.

TIP

In the meantime, here are a few things you can do to implement this philosophy into your life:

>> Believe in the importance of set mealtimes.

>> Make a commitment to follow set mealtimes as much as possible.

- » If you can set up specific mealtimes, do that every morning for the day ahead.

- » Get friends, family, and coworkers involved to help you stick to a plan and eat communally (see the next section).

- » Start slow — even if that means having one set meal on a day off per week. When you see the benefits, you'll be inspired to have more set mealtimes. Every month, add another set mealtime. If your first was Sunday supper, for example, shoot for Saturday lunch as well. Next, start scheduling one meal a day — whether it's breakfast, lunch, or dinner — and make sure you can count on that mealtime to enjoy nourishing yourself.

Making Communal Eating a Priority

"We should look for someone to eat or drink with before looking for something to eat or drink."

—Epicurus

The long history of proverbs relating to the importance of eating together in the Mediterranean region spans from Ancient Egypt to classical Greece to biblical texts, through the Islamic Age of Enlightenment and the Renaissance, and into modern times. Whenever various cultural groups and time periods echo the same pearls of wisdom, it's important to take note. The Mediterranean Diet Pyramid (see Chapter 13) lists eating communally at its base — giving it higher priority in the diet than food itself. It has been proven that eating communally helps children perform better in school, and it helps adults just as much.

According to a popular Italian proverb, "Who eats alone strangles himself in loneliness." This is a practice that everyone in the Mediterranean region lives out on a daily basis. If you've ever been to Cairo, Jerusalem, Palermo, Beirut, or Casablanca and tried to dine alone anywhere other than an airport or major hotel, you'll probably have experienced strangers or restaurant staff coming to sit with you. This is because, throughout the Mediterranean region, it's believed that the company one keeps during a meal is every bit as important as the meal itself. Most people wouldn't allow someone to eat alone, just as they wouldn't serve you a meal without a drink or utensils. This is a deeply engrained aspect of the culture that people who have never lived outside of it take for granted.

According to a study that appeared in the *Journal of Adolescent Health* and was based on interviews with more than 18,000 adolescents, even teenagers who ate regularly with their parents developed much better nutritional habits. Cornell University research also revealed that coworkers of diverse backgrounds who ate together performed better at work. They found that "companies that invest in an inviting cafeteria or shared meal space may be getting a particularly good return on their investment."

Additional surveys show that nearly half of all meals in the United States are eaten alone. Eating alone occasionally *can* be part of a healthful lifestyle, and it can also be enjoyed and even celebrated! When it happens on a regular basis, however, it can take a toll on both mental and physical health. At best, regularly eating alone won't harm you, but it also won't give you any of the additional psychological and physical rewards that eating communally does.

According to MDLinx, a news service for physicians, "The newest epidemic in America [loneliness] now affects up to 47% of adults — double the number affected a few decades ago." The easiest way to fix this is with communal eating. According to *Brain Health*,

> . . . communal eating not only activates beneficial neurochemicals, but also improves digestion. The dining table provides an opportunity for conversation, storytelling, and reconnection. When you bond with others and experience a sense of connection, endogenous opioids and oxytocin [pain- and stress-relieving hormones] are released that stimulate pleasant feelings. The neurochemical changes lead to improved well-being and contentedness.

In a world where stress, loneliness, and depression are consistently on the rise, eating together can be a conscious and deliberate act made to enjoy both pleasure and health at the same time.

Here are my suggestions for making communal eating a part of your life, even if you live alone:

>> Recognize the psychological and health benefits of eating communally.

>> Commit to eating communally some of the time, until it becomes a habit.

>> Schedule breakfast, lunch, or dinner with people whose company you enjoy.

>> Break the rules of who gets to eat together! You don't have to be married or in a romantic relationship or part of a family member to enjoy regular meals together, nor do you need to make a meal a date. You can have eating partners just as you have running or tennis partners and people you carpool with.

» Challenge your preconceived ideas of what can be eaten communally. Many people feel that unless they're eating a really nice meal, it's better to eat alone, but this couldn't be farther from the truth. You'll gain health benefits by eating with others, regardless of what you eat.

» Set up communal eating schedules with coworkers if possible.

» If you must eat alone often, let technology be your friend. Try having a video call with someone at mealtime — you can let them know the health benefits and why you're starting this tradition. It may seem weird at first, so you can try it with coffee or tea. I often tell new friends, "I'll make coffee and then call you." They enjoy the touch of ceremony that it adds to our conversation. After a while "eating together" virtually becomes easier, and your brain gets the psychological benefits of having someone to dine with.

» Begin a food journal and write down who you're going to eat with to emphasize the importance of the new idea.

» Enjoy this opportunity to eat communally. Look at it as a way to get more out of life, invest in your health, and enjoy yourself more.

Chapter **6**

Laughing at Everyday Life

The phrase "Laughter is the best medicine" has been used for millennia. Even the Old Testament discusses the importance of a "merry heart." The 14th-century French surgeon Henri de Mondeville prescribed humor therapy in postoperative treatment plans. It's no surprise then that, in the Mediterranean region, people place a lot of emphasis on humor and laughter. In the Mediterranean, people go to great lengths to make others laugh, put a smile on someone's face, and find the humor in life. Doing so is one of those intangible acts of culture that is hard to explain but definitely worth mentioning because it plays a role in health and happiness. But just how good for you *is* laughter, and why should you make time for something so seemingly trivial?

In this chapter, I explain why laughter is good for you and offer some typical Mediterranean approaches to comic relief, as well as easy ways you can implement them in your life today.

Laughing at Life: Looking at the Research

Taking things seriously has its advantages: It helps you focus, concentrate, and prioritize. But unnecessary stress and worry can occur when you aren't able to laugh at life. When you do make an effort to enjoy humor, you'll treat your mind and body to additional benefits. Nothing works faster than laughter to bring the mind, body, and spirit back into balance than laughter. Taking life less seriously lessens your troubles and enables you to be more hopeful, connected to others, and alert.

In the Mediterranean region, I've heard people say, "Take yourself lightly, take life seriously." Doctors also agree that this strategy works. A good laugh has great short-term and long-term effects. When you start to laugh, it doesn't just lighten your load mentally; it actually induces physical changes in your body. Here's how:

>> Laughing strengthens the immune system.

>> Laughing boosts mood.

>> Laughing diminishes pain and protects the body from the harmful effects of stress.

>> Laughing increases oxygen intake, which stimulates organs such as the heart and lungs.

>> Laughing fires up and quickly relieves your stress response.

>> Laughing stimulates circulation, which helps muscles to relax. In fact, muscles stay relaxed for 45 minutes after a good laugh!

>> Laughing reduces blood pressure. High blood pressure is one of the world's largest health problems and a very dangerous side effect of stress. It puts you at risk for heart disease and stroke. The American Heart Association conducted a study that exposed 79 participants to laughter therapy, which was stimulated through "playful eye contact" and breathing exercises; immediately after these sessions, the blood pressure readings from the laughers lowered significantly, and they continued to have lower blood pressure readings after the three-month study concluded.

>> Laughing helps you to release anger and forgive others more quickly.

>> Laughing triggers *endorphins* (chemicals that boost pleasure and decrease pain), which enhances a sense of well-being and can even lessen or eliminate pain.

>> Laughing helps to increase blood flow, which can help prevent heart disease and cardiovascular issues.

>> Laughing burns some calories. Laughing for 10 to 15 minutes a day can burn approximately 40 calories. In a year's time, that could lead to losing a few pounds!

>> Laughing helps people with cancer live longer than those who don't laugh as much.

With so many health benefits to gain by laughing, it should be at the top of everyone's daily to-do list. The following sections cover a few of the many impressive medical findings about laughter and how it helps specifically with lowering blood pressure and weight loss.

Bringing More Laughter into Your Daily Life

I've spent decades documenting the various ways in which comic relief is put to good use in places like Egypt, Greece, Italy, Lebanon, Morocco, Turkey, and the rest of the region. After referencing many of these occasions countless times, I created some go-to techniques that people around the world can use to brighten their days and lighten their emotional load. Looking for excuses to feel good can create a powerful positive shift in your overall health. These strategies can help you to not only keep stress at bay, but feel better in the process.

Looking for things to laugh at

TIP

In your everyday life, you may not feel like you have much to laugh about. Maybe you're going through a particular stressful situation at work. Maybe you're stressed about money. Or maybe you're living through a pandemic (ahem). When you can't find things in your immediate environment to laugh about, try these techniques:

>> **Watch a favorite comedic movie or a video of your favorite standup comedian.** Don't have any favorite? Ask your family and friends who they like!

>> **Make a collection of memes from social media that you find funny and save them.** Look at them a few times a day or when you need a laugh.

>> **Watch YouTube videos of people laughing.** Years ago, I was diagnosed with a disabling illness. During my treatment, my mind-body therapist suggested I listen to these videos. She said that, like yawning, laughter is contagious, and an important part of healing. Even though it sounded weird, I did what she said, and I found it very helpful!

>> **Keep a journal of the funniest things you've ever heard. Reread** them when you need a laugh.

>> **Designate a comedy buddy and spend time making each other laugh every day.** You don't need to be happy to make jokes. You can make jokes or make your friend laugh because you want to make your friend happy. In return, you laugh, too!

TIP

When you have a hard time lightening up on a topic, try the following:

>> Look at everything with a humorous eye, as if it were a challenge or a job. This lightens situations and helps you let go of resentment.

>> Give others the benefit of the doubt. Before taking offense at something, check to see whether the person meant it in jest.

>> Challenge yourself to see how much you can laugh each day.

Looking for excuses to feel good

Sometimes, after long periods of stress, our bodies and minds can get so used to suffering, that suffering actually feels *normal.* It's easy to forget that feeling good is your natural state — not something you can only achieve on occasion. Vacations, celebrations, and other special occasions shouldn't be the only time you feel good. Those should be the times when you feel good in new places or because you're celebrating a specific event.

Feeling good should be something you aim for on a daily basis. You don't need an excuse or permission from anyone. In the Mediterranean, this is the way in which you give thanks, give back, and contribute — by feeling good as much of the time as possible. For that reason, you rarely find people in the Mediterranean region complaining in public about the way they feel.

In fact, many people take their bodies' clues as a sign that they need to make a conscious effort to feel better more often. When they realize that they aren't mentally or physically aligned, people in the Mediterranean region make a plan — including everything from eating better food to getting better sleep, getting more physical activity, engaging in enjoyable pastimes, socializing more with friends, and getting more sunlight.

TIP

Every morning when you wake up, try asking yourself, "How can I feel better today?" Then, throughout the day, say to yourself "I look for reasons to feel good, and I find them." Say it and think it often. Look forward to good foods, activities, thoughts, and events. You can even keep a journal of the great things that start happening to you as a result. Best of all, if you have an arsenal of healthful foods, thoughts, things to do, and so on, that make you feel good, you'll be able to improve both your mental and physical health greatly.

It can be really helpful to write down or keep a list of all the things that make you feel the best — and the lightest. Whether it's butterflies, a lighthearted song, a fond memory, a video, a piece of music . . . it makes no difference. The main point is that you have a stash of go-to topics, thoughts, and things to turn to when you want to feel better. Use any excuse, as many people in the Mediterranean region do, to feel good!

The good news is: Laughter is a free tool within everyone's reach. You use it to support your emotional and mental health every day. Laughing more often leads to better relationships and longevity. In the Mediterranean region, taking the time and making the effort to make someone laugh shows care and concern. Try making a conscious effort to laugh more and to put a smile on the face of others more often while looking for more excuses to feel good and note the positive changes that you experience while doing so.

BLUE ZONE SECRETS

Blue Zones are regions of the world where a higher than usual number of people live much longer and better than average. The term first appeared in Dan Buettner's November 2005 *National Geographic* cover story, "The Secrets of a Long Life." Not all Mediterranean countries are Blue Zones — only the islands of Sardinia and Ikaria are — but the Blue Zone ideal applies to what takes place on a daily basis in many places in the Mediterranean.

I told one of my Greek friends that I was planning on spending time on the island of Ikaria ("the land where people forget to die"), and I talked all about the Blue Zone mentality and what I hoped to learn while I was there. He chuckled to himself and said, "Amy, those people live forever and are healthy because they don't give a damn." And he continued laughing. In the United States, we talk a lot about being able to "let go" of our problems. But my friend, in his lighthearted way, reminded me that sometimes it's healthiest not to "pick up" problems to begin with — so you don't have to "let go." Certain places just seem more laid back, and their residents don't feel the need to stress out.

Chapter **7**

Participating in Pleasurable Activity

The base of the Mediterranean Diet Pyramid (see Chapter 13) highlights the importance of physical activity. You don't have to spend hours grinding away at a gym or working out with machines, however, to enjoy better health. In this chapter, I introduce pleasurable, Mediterranean ways to stay fit and enjoy yourself in the process.

Doing What You Love

All activity can be beneficial, for a variety of reasons, but certain ones have the power to keep the mind, body, and spirit healthy. Doing what you love is one of the greatest joys in life. Those good feelings translate into less stress and pain, as well as more enjoyment and good health.

I've enjoyed the pleasures of baking, cooking, reading, and writing since I was three years old. Those are the activities that *I* enjoy doing the most, so I know they're good for me. The trick is to find the activities *you* enjoy doing. Maybe you love gardening or woodworking or knitting.

We have no control over many aspects of our lives. But there are some things we *can* control, and that's where the art of everyday living comes into play. Our thoughts, how we feed ourselves, how we dress, how we choose to feel, and so on are things that are usually within our control. It's no coincidence that most people in the Mediterranean region try to enjoy those aspects of life the most. By preparing the best possible meals for themselves, they at least know that they'll get pleasure during those times of the day when they cook and eat.

The joy of cooking

Cooking is a daily escape for many people all over the world. In addition to the psychological and physical benefits of cooking, our bodies actually eat less food and absorb more nutrients when we simply smell foods cooking prior to eating them.

Depending upon the amount of effort you put into it, and the exact activity, cooking can burn between 143 and 415 calories per hour. On the higher end of that scale, that may be about what you would burn while walking briskly for the same amount of time. For me, the additional pleasure that I feel while cooking, the sense of purpose I have, and the creative outlet it provides all make cooking a great exercise!

The mental health benefits associated with baking bread — such as kneading the dough and getting it into the right shape — can help relieve tension. Plus, the process of patiently waiting for the bread to rise over the course of a couple of hours can help you feel a sense of delayed gratification.

Psychologists believe that cooking and baking are therapeutic because they cause *behavioral activation,* a type of therapy that alleviates depression, anxiety, and attention deficit hyperactivity disorder (ADHD) by increasing goal-oriented behavior and preventing procrastination. The sense of control is mentally empowering. Cooking and baking require constant focused attention on each step of preparation. Jokingly called "tasty meditation" by many, they've been proven to provide calming, creative, and soothing effects on those who choose to submit to their charms.

Best of all, you can get these same benefits even if you're cooking by and for yourself. When you cook with and for others, though, you get the additional benefit of community connections, a sense of service, and the positive emotions associated with the sense of giving. Our primal instincts are always calmed when we nourish ourselves and others. *Psychology Today* magazine even cited cooking as a great source of mindful therapy, which also provides sensory pleasure.

When we re-create old family (or other) recipes, we're also connecting to the past in a positive way, which is an important factor in mental health. Some therapists are even holding sessions in the kitchen because they're finding that cognitive-behavioral therapy can be extremely effective. In my own life, something about the act of cooking and baking — and the mundane tasks that give you something to focus on — helps people to open up in an easy and natural way. I notice this the most with children and young adults. Often when you ask kids about their lives, they respond quickly and say there's nothing new or nothing bothering them. But when they're working in the kitchen, without even being prompted, I find that kids (and many times adults) really open up.

After years of witnessing children, adults, and professional chefs share and work through some of their biggest obstacles to happiness in the kitchen with me, I've come to some of my own conclusions:

>> **People are usually comfortable in the kitchen.** Something about all our senses being activated in a place where many of us have fond memories of a relative or caregiver making nourishing food for us makes us feel at ease.

>> **Being around a stove takes the pressure off.** When you're busy doing an activity, it takes the pressure off of being right and making sense, so opening up seems less intimidating. Plus, because there's a lot going on in the kitchen, letting your guard down is easy because if the conversation starts going in a place that makes you uncomfortable, there are distractions to help you get back on track again.

The kitchen has become a bonding place for me, my friends, and my loved ones in a much deeper way than I could ever have imagined. Nowadays instead of saying "Let's talk," I'm more likely to say, "Let's cook" or "Let's bake." For the people I share professional kitchens with, I don't even need to do that, because I know that whatever we need to work out will surface naturally. The great cookbook author and restaurateur Lidia Bastianich once said that cooks don't go to therapists. When something is bothering them, they head to the kitchen and bang things out until they feel better. I believe in the need for and efficacy of a trained therapist, but I do know exactly what Lidia meant — and I, too, head to the kitchen when I need to feel better.

The pleasure principle

The activities that we enjoy the most are the best for us. According to research, it's in our best interest to do more of what we love. All types of hobbies have physical and mental health benefits? Dancing, gardening, running, baking — it doesn't matter whether your chosen pastime is low impact or highly active, doing what you love can reduce stress, broaden your social circle, lift your spirits, reduce chronic pain, and add quality to your life.

Different types of stress require different types of activities to feel better, but what you enjoy the most will be most beneficial. Your favorite physical activity — whether it's shooting hoops, running, jogging, playing tennis, swimming, or kickboxing — can be effective in lowering your heart rate, improving your mood, and reducing stress.

Even less strenuous activities, such as knitting, painting, sewing, gardening, petting your favorite furry friend, or reading a book can improve your health, as long as you enjoy what you're doing. Many people have meaningful pastimes, hobbies, and even careers that haven't always appealed to them. I have friends who've taken art courses on a dare, thinking they would hate it, only to later go on to win awards and open galleries to showcase their creations — so don't rule anything out!

It doesn't matter whether you're singing, dancing, biking, or cooking, if your passions include physical activity, you're doing your our minds and bodies a big favor. Pleasurable activities reduce your risk of heart disease, diabetes, cancer, and inflammation (which is at the base of all diseases). Less than an hour of physical activity each week can reduce your risk of premature death by more than 18 percent. If we get two and a half hours (a bit more than 20 minutes a day) of moderately intense physical activity every week, that same risk is reduced to 31 percent!

REMEMBER

No one in the Mediterranean region is counting minutes of exercise. Traditionally, people do what makes them feel the best simply for that reason and with the innate knowledge that they deserve to feel good, and that what they enjoy the most is best for them.

TIP

Here are a few ways to get more pleasurable activities in your life:

>> Acknowledge the health benefits to doing the things you love most and make them a priority.

>> Join a group — a sports league, baking club, or volunteer organization.

>> Take note of any activities you have to do (like cleaning the house or mowing the lawn) and brainstorm ways to enjoy yourself doing them more.

>> Review your bucket list and make a plan to start doing one of the things on that list as soon as possible.

>> Practice Pilates or yoga.

>> Swim laps in a pool.

>> Go for a walk in a park around your neighborhood or workplace.

>> Take a class on a topic you're interested in.

>> Read about subjects you've always been curious about.

If you're at a loss for where to start, think about the things that have given you the most pleasure in the past and decide whether they're worth repeating. If those activities don't appeal to you right now, be open to new ones. Try new things out with friends and envision yourself enjoying doing something different. Discovering a new joy, just like a new dish, can do great things for human happiness.

Hobbies and a sense of purpose

Many people take hobbies for granted. Some even consider pastimes to be nothing more than things we do when we're bored.

When I was in college, I began to appreciate hobbies from a deeper sense. I was in treatment for chronic neck and back pain. The therapist told me I held tension in a particular area and gave me treatments to heal it. One day, in the middle of a session, she asked whether I did anything I enjoyed in which I wasn't evaluated, judged, or watched. At first, I didn't even know what she was talking about, but she explained how participating in activities that I could do just for the pure *fun* of it — without expecting or needing anything to come from it — could be very beneficial. I honestly couldn't think of anything at first, but then I remembered baking.

Having a sense of purpose is one of the most important common denominators among the healthiest cultures in the Mediterranean. Figuring out our role in the universe was the eternal quest of the ancients, and embracing the wisdom in this quest provides great satisfaction and a healthy mental outlook in the modern world, too. In various Mediterranean countries, people adopt a philosophical or religious outlook that pertains to their own cultures. The particular credo, if they truly believe and embrace it, can bring them comfort and joy.

A study conducted at the University of California, San Diego, in 2020 suggested that having purpose in life makes you more likely to feel better both mentally and physically. More than 1,000 adults ranging in age from 21 to older than 100 were surveyed using questionnaires designed to analyze their physical and mental well-being. Additional questionnaires researched the degree to which the adults found meaning in their lives. The studies revealed that people who perceived that they had found meanings in their lives felt mentally and physically better than those who did not (this was especially true for the older study participants).

Unlike cultures in the Mediterranean, the culture of the United States doesn't reinforce particular religious or cultural credos. One of the advantages of our diversity is that we can know and learn from others around us. This often causes us to question our identities and to feel a need to discover them on our own, whereas people in more homogenous societies in the Mediterranean often take their own culture's philosophy for granted. In the United States, we usually aren't true cultural natives; instead, we have access to countless creeds and philosophies. It's up to us to incorporate the inspiration from our ancestors along with new approaches that may appeal to us in order to come up with a way of thinking and believing that complements our spirits as well as our minds and bodies.

REMEMBER

The comforting aspect of finding purpose to your life is accepted by doctors as having a positive effect on physical health. But this doesn't mean that if you don't have a lofty purpose that you can't achieve great health. Sometimes people don't even think about their life's purpose until they're faced with a major crisis or life-threatening illness, so if you aren't bothered by the thought of not having a sense of purpose, you don't need to worry about it now.

Other health professionals believe that enjoyable leisure activities are associated with psychological and physical well-being. After all, achieving optimal health is an accomplishment that is, in itself, important and essential.

Certain types of hobbies — present in both the Mediterranean and the United States — help to boost the brain by stimulating and challenging the mind. The arts are especially effective at this. Calligraphy, drawing, poetry, songwriting, listening to music, attending theatrical events, and visiting art museums are all pleasurable hobbies that can help your mental strength. Nowadays, fortunately, you don't even have to go far to access a lot of these creative outlets — classes, videos, and entire library and museum collections are available online! These types of activities enhance not only creativity, but your sense of focus as well. Just 8½ hours per month (that's a little over 2 hours per week) of activities like these can improve your mental health and confidence levels significantly.

Learning a new language, writing, designing websites, woodworking, homebrewing, winemaking, cooking, ceramics, and taking classes on topics you love are also good for your health. You may feel like you can't afford to do certain activities, both in terms of time and money. But many classes are available for free or quite inexpensively both online and in person nowadays. And if it's time you're short on, when you switch your thought process from seeing hobbies as a luxury to seeing them as a necessity, you often find times for the things you couldn't seem to before. When you realize that these particular types of activities are good for your health, you may find ways to incorporate them in your daily life.

DON'T WAIT UNTIL RETIREMENT!

People often talk about what they're going to do when they retire. And for obvious reasons, people can't fit all their bucket list plans into their busy work schedule, but if there's something you've got on hold until retirement, you may feel better doing it now. The things we save to do until retirement are usually the things that appeal to us. Why not infuse them into your life now? Don't put off for retirement what you could be doing today!

When people retire, they often join study groups, start to exercise, take up painting, or discover a new love of the culinary arts. But why wait? You may feel like you don't have the time, so you put off what you could do today until you're totally free in retirement. But you can still get your feet wet with some of these activities. For example, maybe you've always dreamed of spending a summer in the Mediterranean when you retire, but there's no way you have the time or money for that now. Why not take a Mediterranean cooking class? Or sign up for an Italian language course? Or have a Mediterranean movie night once a week where you watch films set in the region? Maybe you could start a group on Meetup (www.meetup.com), where you meet once a month with other people who share your passion.

Enjoying and making the most out of the present while still maintaining and looking forward to achieving positive goals is invigorating and an important element of happiness. Regardless of what you do, positive thoughts and daydreaming can help you bridge the gap between where you are today and where you hope to be tomorrow.

Volunteering for or creating organizations that you believe in is another wonderful way to add healthful, quality time to your schedule. When you volunteer for causes that you believe in, you feel better. The satisfaction of giving back to your community is a powerful form of love that doesn't always get the attention it deserves.

REMEMBER

The mental and physical healing aspects of doing what you enjoy is priceless. Take control of your well-being, and do more of what you enjoy!

Types of Physical Activity in the Mediterranean Lifestyle

The traditional Mediterranean lifestyle offers plenty of ways to stay active without spending money or going to extremes. Some of your most natural and necessary movements can give you the benefits of staying active that you need. No gym membership or in-home equipment? No problem. You can get in shape the way people have done for thousands of years. Looking for inspiration? The DIY attitude toward growing and making your own food and caring for your own home, yard, and garden may be just what the doctor ordered.

Staying fit without the gym

Some people love going to gyms and working out with equipment at home. Good for them! But if you don't find gym workouts enjoyable, that's fine, too. According to the people who live in areas with the highest concentration of centenarians, the physical activity that brings you the most joy will benefit your health the most.

Finding a healthful activity — or two or three or four — that you can do daily can help keep you going strong well into old age. Walking is probably the most common form of exercise in the traditional Mediterranean lifestyle. Whatever activity you do, the goal is to get your entire body moving, work up a sweat, and breathe heavily. Do that five to ten hours a week if you really want to see maximum results.

TIP

If you're committed to walking an hour a day, the walking doesn't need to be done at one time — it could be 30 minutes before breakfast and another 30 minutes after dinner, or 20 minutes after each meal. Maybe you can walk to the grocery store or to run errands — those minutes count, too. Even taking the stairs can be an important part of an exercise program — you may not live in an area with the kinds of hills found in the Mediterranean region (not many people do!), but you can climb stairs and get the same benefits, just without the incredible views.

Bicycling is very popular in the Mediterranean region because it was once the main mode of transportation. Nowadays it's a popular modern sport. Bicycling relieves stress on the joints.

REMEMBER

You don't need to run marathons or overwork your body in order to stay fit. Many people enjoy the thrill and sense of achievement that comes from finishing marathons, but exercising at a pace and in a manner that is kind to the joints is recommended for most people. Tai chi, yoga, swimming, and Pilates, combined with eating nutritious foods, can cause the tissues and cells in the body to repair and heal themselves. Thirty to forty minutes of these activities every other day, in addition to walking or getting other forms of exercise, will provide positive mental and physical benefits for your health.

Adopting a DIY attitude

My maternal grandmother cooked, cleaned, sewed, knitted, crocheted, baked, decorated wedding cakes, painted, made statues, drew, decorated, and repaired things in her home and car. My paternal grandfather tended a garden and made everything from scratch, including wine and spirits. In our world, asking for help and buying things were seen as signs of weakness.

TIP

Now, you don't have to do everything my grandparents did — and I don't either! But you can look for ways to infuse more DIY into your daily life. Start by asking yourself what you enjoy making, and make an effort to do more of that. If you've always wanted to learn a craft, get a book or take a class and learn. Then share the results of your hard work with your loved ones. Next time you visit, you'll be able to bring them a scarf you knitted or beer you brewed yourself!

Whether you begin your own herb garden in a pot, start giving away batches of your favorite cookies to friends, or share your homemade sauce or jewelry with loved ones, you'll be making yourself and others happy. The pleasures of doing the things you enjoy the most for others gives you a sense of satisfaction, and completion. Whatever you choose to make is a creation all your own — the pleasure you derive from it can never be taken from you. When you share these gifts with others, it's as if you're giving them access to your private world, sharing a piece of yourself. It's a win-win situation for everyone involved.

Chapter **8**

Engaging with Nature

M ental health experts recommend 30 minutes of fresh air a day — and many believe it's more beneficial to the psyche than antipsychotic drugs! In this chapter, I explain the research behind spending time in nature, offer fun and creative ways to enjoy more time outdoors, and highlight the importance of spending time in the sun.

Looking at the Research behind the Importance of Nature

Getting more fresh air and spending time outdoors can help to increase your overall health and mental outlook. Increased digestion, better immunity, improved mood, and reduced risk of illness are just a few of the benefits you have to look forward to by spending more time outside. According to one government estimate, the average American spends 90 percent of their life indoors. People in the Mediterranean region, however, look for every excuse they can to be outside.

Even when I try to plan outdoor activities with many of my friends in the United States, many fears come up — sunburn, flies, mosquitos, ticks. . . . Some worry that it may start to rain.

REMEMBER

Regardless of the risks of the outdoors, the benefits outweigh the risks. Long, loose, light-colored clothing, sunscreen, and bug spray can keep you from getting burned or bitten. But few things provide the benefits that fresh air brings.

Research shows that spending time outdoors leads to more physical exercise, too. A British study of 1,000 children found that they were twice as physically active when they were outside than indoors. When adults make being outdoors a goal, they tend to enjoy walking, doing yard work, biking, gardening, fishing, golfing, and sports more often than when they're indoors.

FRESH AIR

Each year I anticipate the arrival of spring and look forward to opening the window to enjoy the *Sham an Nassim*, the smell of the fresh breeze that the Ancient Egyptians even had a festival for. In fact, many cultures, including the Ancient Persians, celebrated the New Year with the arrival of spring. Some ancient traditions associate the quality of air with divinity itself, and because it's essential to health and well-being, it's no surprise as to why.

I open my windows daily — no matter what the weather — just to get fresh air in the house. I share this custom with many women in the Mediterranean region. Opening the window was a sign of the start of the day — fresh energy, and a time to clean, refresh, and renew. One of the greatest joys is opening the windows in spring when the quality of air has changed to a newer, seemingly fresher quality.

The Sham an Nassim festival in still celebrated in Egypt today. Much of the symbolism behind this ancient holiday inspired today's modern Easter traditions. The celebration began during antiquity, and when Christianity became wide spread, it was held in the middle of the Coptic Lenten period. The Coptic Christians, who were abstaining from meat, fish, dairy products, and sweets for Lent, couldn't participate. Under Fatimid Muslim rule in the 10th century, the date was changed so that everyone could participate in the festivities. The Fatimids changed the date to Coptic Easter Monday, so that the festival would still be in springtime, but after the Lenten fasting period was over.

Because the holiday has no religious connotations, Egyptians of all faiths celebrated with picnics, outings, and family gatherings. Each menu item was symbolically important. Fresh sardines and fish in general, were symbols of fertility, and they were available to commoners and pharaohs alike. The fish were also symbolic because Ancient Egyptians would make offerings of fish to the gods during holidays and then fast. They would salt cure and marinate the fish to enjoy after the day's fasting.

Fast-forward thousands of years and our access to fresh air still deserves to be enjoyed and celebrated. Every breath we take is a luxury that shouldn't be taken for granted. Our mental and physical health depend on it, and getting more of it increases both.

Light elevates people's moods, so being outdoors can lead to more positive emotions, laughter, and mental well-being. In 2010, English scientists reported that just five minutes of exercise in open, green spaces resulted in improvements in both self-esteem and mood.

Nature-deficit disorder was a term coined in 2018 to support the theory that children with attention deficit hyperactivity disorder (ADHD) focused better after being outdoors. In 2008, studies revealed that they scored better on concentration tests if they walked through a park rather than a neighborhood or downtown area. People with ADHD also show positive results after exercising outdoors. Regardless of your age, the greener the outdoor access, the more your concentration will improve.

Natural light also helps people to heal faster. University of Pittsburgh researchers found that spinal surgery patients suffered less pain and stress and took fewer pain medications during their recoveries when they were exposed to natural light. Hospital studies have shown that patients with a view of trees outside their windows recovered better than those staring at a brick wall, and when the additional benefit of fresh air was added, the results were even better.

Carving Out Time to Spend in Nature

You may already be living the busiest lives imaginable — maybe you're even busier than you've ever been. The thought of adding something new into your schedule or doing things differently can be daunting. If the idea of adding something else to your life makes you feel more stressed, then it may be a good idea to wait a bit and revisit the idea at a calmer time. But if you're inspired to spend more time in nature and get more fresh air because you're convinced that it will help you, that's a different story.

REMEMBER

People in the Mediterranean region and around the world have important things to do, too. They just value their own health and well-being and know that spending time in nature enables them to take advantage of free nutrients and health benefits that we were designed to enjoy as humans.

TIP

There are several easy changes you can make that will have large combined pay-offs and help you enjoy more outdoor time:

>> **Do whatever you've been wanting to do.** Maybe you've been thinking "I want to get outside and plant some flowers." Promise yourself at least five minutes a day doing that. Everyone can afford five minutes, and it can be enough to create positive effects.

>> **Give your indoor time as much "outdoor access" as possible.** For example, rearrange your office so your desk faces a window with greenery instead of away from it. If you don't have a window in your office or area where you spend a lot of time, think about a way in which you can shift your activity around so you can be in front of a window while indoors. Maybe position your kitchen table or living room couch so that you can see out a window.

>> **If there are parks in your area, identify which ones are closest and plan to visit them every week.** You could schedule a long weekend walk at one of them, a 30-minute lunch in another, and a few minutes to breathe deeply, refresh, and renew yourself in another. Or maybe you can do all those things on different days in a different green area (for example, on your terrace or in your backyard).

>> **Take anything that you *can* do outdoors outdoors.** I take my computer to the park with me, or out onto the front porch, or into the backyard, or to outdoor cafes. I love to walk and run and eat and socialize in all those places, too. But if I'm on a deadline and I have the choice of writing indoors or out, and the weather is obliging, guess which one I choose?

REMEMBER

No matter what kind of work you do, spending time outdoors will inspire you. You may have noticed that some of your best ideas or solutions to problems came to you while you were in nature. Access to nature is probably one of the most underestimated health resources of modern times. Luckily, nature is all around!

Getting Enough Time in the Sun

Something about the word *Mediterranean* conjures up images of the sun. Mother Nature did bestow relatively mild climatic conditions on the region, but the weather isn't always perfect there. Did you know that Washington, DC, actually averages four more hours of sunlight per year than Barcelona does? And although Athens and Nice get a few hundred more hours of sunshine every year, Istanbul and Naples actually get *less* sunlight than Washington, DC.

What that means is you can't use weather or geographic conditions as an excuse not to incorporate Mediterranean-style living in the United States. If Washington, DC, gets the same amount of sun as Barcelona, then we should start celebrating the sun the way the Spaniards do! Those who live in the Mediterranean region take advantage of every bit of sunshine they can get to spend outdoors.

A SUNNY DISPOSITION

Spend a significant amount of time around people speaking Italian, and you'll hear the word *solare,* which means "sunny." If an Italian tells you *sei solare* ("you're sunny"), it's one of the greatest compliments they can give you. Other compliments like *sei il mio sole* ("you are my sun") can be heard in Italian poetry and love songs. What could be a better compliment to someone than comparing them to the ultimate source of light, warmth, and happiness? Being *solare,* or having a sunny disposition, is truly something that people in the region, and especially in Italy, aspire to. A smile, a happy thought, a kind word, bright colors, a warm embrace, and positivity are all associated with someone who is *solare,* and Italians try their best to demonstrate and appreciate these qualities as much as possible.

To have a sunny disposition is to be an optimist. People in the Mediterranean region tend to be highly optimistic as a whole. This doesn't mean that they're Pollyannas or that they don't live in the real world. It just means that, given the choice of looking on the bright side or wallowing in self-pity and sorrow, they usually choose the former. In Italian, there is an expression *Alla vita tu sorridi, e la vita ti sorriderà,* which means "If you smile at life, life will smile at you." In addition to saying that phrase, most people demonstrate it in their daily lives.

Part of having a sunny disposition is learning not only to withstand the storms, but to learn to dance in them, and people in the Mediterranean region have embraced that mentality.

The sense of community that exists in many places in the region also helps people to have a sunny disposition. Happiness is contagious. When we're in groups that want to have fun and enjoy life, it often doesn't leave room for worrying, complaining, or pointing out everything that's wrong or missing from a situation. Living in a community like that makes it difficult to feel bad. If you were to confide in a loved one about something negative that you were experiencing, they would try their best to help you, and if they couldn't, they would do their best to take your mind off the problem and distract you with something pleasurable.

A sunny disposition isn't considered fake or phony in the Mediterranean. Instead, it's considered the result of a person who cared enough about themselves and others to put their best face forward.

A cheerful attitude can even help you live longer. Johns Hopkins University researchers conducted a 25-year study on the topic and found that feeling optimistic, cheerful, and energetic about life reduced your risk of suffering a heart attack. Their findings even showed that those with a high risk of developing coronary artery disease due to their family histories were still half as likely to develop it because of their sunny disposition.

(continued)

(continued)

Speaking of family history, we may learn optimism and pessimism from our parents. If negativity seems to run in your family, you'll be doing yourself a favor by using whatever method works for you to change the cycle. One large study of 2,300 older adults over two years found that those who were more positive had a greater likelihood of staying healthy and living independently than their pessimistic peers.

In the 1960s, research done over a 30-year period found that optimism was linked to a better outcome on eight measures of physical and mental function and health. In similar studies, the mortality rate among pessimists rose by 19 percent. Another study conducted on University of North Carolina students over a 40-year period found that those who were pessimistic had a 42 percent higher rate of death than their optimistic classmates during that time period, with cancer being the most common.

One of the silent causes of many of our illnesses is the constant high levels of the stress hormone cortisol. Studies have shown that a positive attitude was linked to lower levels of cortisol despite the various demographics of the research participants. Two additional markers of inflammation (C-reactive protein and interleukin-6) were also found to be lower in women with sunnier dispositions. These two components help reduce risk of heart attack and stroke, reduce the levels of adrenaline, and improve immunity.

Moods and overall satisfaction of life have very positive effects on well-being. People with anxiety and depression have proven to live shorter lives than those who have a happy outlook. As modern research continues to explore the benefits of a sound mind–body connection, the age-old Italian adage of "healthy mind, healthy body" still rings true.

What the research says about sunlight

Soaking up the sun provides us with positive emotions, increased vitamin D, better immunity, stronger bones, better skin, and more. Exposure to sunlight helps to increase levels of the hormone serotonin in our brains. Serotonin helps us to feel calm and to focus while preventing or reducing stress, depression, anxiety, panic attacks, and premenstrual dysphoric disorder.

When sunlight enters the eyes, serotonin is triggered in special places in the retina. For this reason, light therapy is often prescribed for people with depression, and light therapy boxes (which mimic sunlight) are available for this purpose. Of course, good old–fashioned sunlight is the best option.

Many people avoid sunlight altogether because they're afraid of skin cancer, but a moderate amount of sun exposure also has preventive benefits. People who live in areas with fewer daylight hours have a higher incidence of colon, ovarian, pancreatic, prostrate, and other cancers than those who live in sunny areas.

The World Health Organization recognizes sun exposure as a treatment to help people with skin conditions such as psoriasis, eczema, jaundice, and acne. Irritable bowel disease, rheumatoid arthritis, thyroiditis, lupus, and other conditions have a tendency to benefit from increased sun exposure as well. Many modern doctors are beginning to suggest that avoiding the sun completely has very negative effects on our health.

Researchers in Spain found that children who have regular access to sunshine have a lower incidence of respiratory diseases, like asthma, than those who did not. Improved lung health is credited to the sun's natural abundance of immune-protective vitamin D — commonly found in lower levels in children with asthma.

Getting enough vitamin D helps you to be less susceptible to fractures and reduces inflammation (which is at the base of all disease and pain. The sunshine vitamin has also proven effective in preventing diabetes because vitamin D is needed to make and secrete insulin.

The essential vitamin also helps reduce blood pressure and the risk of hypertension and builds stronger muscles. One often overlooked benefit of vitamin D is that it decreases certain respiratory and food allergies. Those who suffer from celiac disease, asthma, and psoriasis should rule out vitamin D deficiencies before being diagnosed.

Vitamin D also improves energy and enhances mood. Because most cells in our bodies contain vitamin D receptors, cells with access to the nutrient perform their best. This includes lowering the risk of cognitive diseases such as Alzheimer's disease, dementia, and autism.

One of my other happiest discoveries was learning that the sun may help slow weight gain and balance blood sugar. The University of Edinburgh published research that suggests that moderate sun exposure can help slow weight gain and prevent diabetes. In this particular study, the beneficial effects of the UV light weren't the result of increased vitamin D levels as is usually the case. Instead, it came from nitric oxide — a compound naturally produced in the skin following sun exposure.

Some special medical attention was given to early morning light in a study from Northwestern University, which proved that those exposed to sunlight between 8 a.m. and noon had lower body mass indexes (BMIs) than those who were exposed to the sun later in the day. This is because our natural circadian clocks, which play a role in our sleep quality, energy, blood sugar, weight, and hormones, benefit from early morning light.

The truth about vitamin D

My good friend, culinary medicine partner, and co-creator of @culinarymedlife, Dr. Sam Pappas, was the first person to effectively explain to me, and our audiences, the importance of vitamin D and the often overlooked role it plays in our immune system. During the COVID-19 pandemic, vitamin D proved to be increasingly important in our immunity, but understanding and using it properly can be complicated.

Not all types of "the sunshine vitamin" are created equal. The way in which the body absorbs vitamin D varies, so it's important to learn more about the topic before randomly popping pills or sleeping in the sun.

Increased exposure to the sun will help your vitamin D levels to rise. When the skin is exposed to the sun, the liver and kidneys begin to create a biologically active form of vitamin D. Unlike many other vitamins, vitamin D has been proven to have disease-fighting potential. Studies have shown that vitamin D can help to prevent strokes, heart attacks, osteoporosis, rickets, bone diseases, cancer, and depression.

Most Americans would be considered vitamin D deficient, especially by Mediterranean standards, because we don't consume as much vitamin D in our food, and we don't spend as much time in the sun. Doctors believe that we can make all the vitamin D we need by getting outdoors more often. Exposing our arms and legs for just 15 minutes every sunny day can help.

REMEMBER

Not all people produce the same amounts of vitamin D. By age 65, for example, our bodies produce about 25 percent of the amount that they did when we were in our twenties. Skin color also plays a role in vitamin D absorption. African Americans have half the amount of vitamin D in their blood that Caucasian Americans do. Ask your doctor to test your vitamin D levels (with a simple blood test) to ensure you're getting enough. The optimal blood level of vitamin D is not concretely established but likely falls between 20 and 50 ng/mL.

Stress, medications, and other health conditions can also play a role in decreasing the amount of Vitamin D that our bodies make on their own. Sunscreen, which blocks UVB light, can also block vitamin D production. There is a lot of controversy surrounding sunscreen and vitamin D in the United States, but it's generally accepted that limited yet focused sun exposure supplemented with vitamin D pills can be an effective way of creating some natural vitamin D without risking sun damage.

TIP

If you have concerns about your sun exposure and vitamin D levels, talk with your doctor.

Easy ways to get more of "the sun vitamin"

One study found that in a 30-minute period while wearing a swimsuit, most Caucasian people produced 50,000 international units (IUs) of vitamin D, while those with tanned skin produced 20,000 to 30,000 IUs and dark-skinned people produced 8,000 to 10,000 IUs. Be sure to evaluate your sun exposure and the vitamin D found in your blood and come up with a plan with your healthcare provider to ensure that you're getting enough.

Vitamin D can be found in some foods, including fatty fish (such as herring, mackerel, salmon, and sardines) and cod liver oil. Eggs and caviar also contain some vitamin D. Mushrooms contain a pro-vitamin called ergosterol, which is converted into vitamin D. (The mushrooms absorb vitamin D in a similar manner to humans. If mushrooms are grown while exposed to UV lamps, they're labeled "UV-treated" or "high in vitamin D" and contain 400 IU of the nutrient per 3 ounces.) Even one serving of liver, though not a favorite of many people, contains about 12 percent of the necessary daily requirement of vitamin D.

In the United States, vitamin D is frequently added to dairy products (such as milk and yogurt), orange juice, and soy. Because those methods aren't natural and can offer varying results, traditional Mediterranean habits would prefer vitamin D to be gained from exposure to sunlight. Supplements are a good addition when deemed necessary by a medical professional, though.

Easy ways to increase your vitamin D levels, in addition to getting more sun exposure, include:

>> **Cod liver oil:** A tablespoon of cod liver oil contains 1,360 IU of vitamin D.

>> **Supplements:** High-quality vitamin D3 supplements (which come from animal sources) or vitamin D2 supplements (which comes from plant sources) are two options.

>> **UV lamps:** UV lamps that emit UV-B radiation may boost vitamin D levels. UV lamps mimic the action of the sun and can be especially helpful if your sun exposure is limited due to your location or inability to go outdoors, but they shouldn't be used for more than 15 minutes at a time.

Different people require different amounts of vitamin D, but typically 1,000 to 4,000 IU is considered a safe daily dose for maintaining healthy levels of vitamin D. Those suffering with chronic illnesses or dealing with other factors may require higher doses. Vitamin C and calcium supplementation can be important to ensure absorption of vitamin D.

Talk to your doctor about how much vitamin D to take. In the United States, various sources state that adults require different amounts:

- **Endocrine Society:** 1,500 to 2,000 IU

- **Reference Daily Intake (RDI):** 600 to 800 IU

- **U.S. National Academy of Medicine:** 600 to 800 IU

Daily consumption of more than 4,000 IU is not recommended and may be toxic to the body.

MAKING THE BEST OF IT

Ancient cultures in the Mediterranean basin know and realize the perils of adversity first hand. The general attitude in the region is that it's bad enough that we have to experience certain unpleasantries in life. There are certain things that are out of our control and that we don't like. Because there is nothing we can do to change them, however, we focus our attention instead on the things that we love, on what we're grateful for, on what inspires us, and, of course, what we can change.

In addition, regardless of the particular Mediterranean culture or community, people have learned to make the best of it. They're so used to thriving in less-than-perfect situations that they can create masterpieces often out of very little.

I remember when I was a little girl, I used to cook with my grandfather. He had vivid memories of being a cook in the military during World War II, so he wanted me to be able to make the most out of what I had on hand. Even though we had access to a lot of ingredients and could afford them, he would always make me cook with leftovers or subpar goods, or replace a necessary ingredient in a recipe with a whole coconut, for example. He wanted to stretch my imagination and make me be resourceful.

I didn't appreciate his tactics when I was 4 years old, but today I pride myself on being one of the most resourceful chefs around. Many of my assistants ask how I can keep my calm in stressful situations and why I'm such a low-maintenance cook. I tell them the story of my grandfather, as well as other less-than-perfect conditions I've cooked in around the world, and then they understand.

Even if you have unlimited resources and things are seemingly in control, so many forces in the universe are beyond our control that being resourceful is still a great skill to develop. It makes you feel more creative, enables you to solve problems, and helps you to not sweat the small stuff.

Chapter **9**

Setting Aside Time for Siestas

Although the ritual of an afternoon siesta is rooted in Spain, where it's still widely practiced, these afternoon breaks are sacred across the Mediterranean region, even in large cities such as Athens and Tel Aviv.

TECHNICAL STUFF

The word *siesta* comes from the Latin *hora sexta*, which means "the sixth hour" and refers to when the calendars were divided into 12-hour days during Roman times. Spain introduced the siesta centuries ago, supposedly to provide their farmers with a time to rest during the hottest time of the day.

Due to Spain's wide influence, throughout the Mediterranean, the custom of allowing people to sleep though the hottest part of the day and avoid the sun's strong midday rays has expanded. Nowadays, the siesta involves sleeping for about 20 minutes after a meal. Some people nap earlier, others later, and times vary, even by day. The important thing to note is that naps are available to all, and the benefits that they offer are many.

In this chapter, I explain the benefits of napping and show you how you can easily fit naps into your schedule.

THE DIFFERENT KINDS OF NAPS

According to science, not all naps are created equal, and many factors impact how helpful naps can be. It's important to understand your body's own needs when trying to determine the best type of nap for you:

- **Recovery naps** help you to make up for lost sleep at night.

- **Prophylactic naps** are taken to prevent sleep loss. They're often used by night-shift workers before and during their shifts in order to prevent sleepiness and to stay alert while working.

- **Appetitive naps** are taken simply for the pleasure of doing so. They're known to improve mood and energy upon waking.

- **Fulfillment naps** are scheduled for children to ensure that they get enough sleep.

- **Essential naps** are taken when you're healing or fighting off an illness.

This chapter focuses mainly on appetitive naps, which are closest in nature to the siestas of the Mediterranean region. You may hear that a nap time of 10, 20, or 30 minutes is optimal for napping, but what matters is determining what's best for you. You should feel refreshed when waking up from a nap, not groggy. If you're sick or suffering from an illness, you may require longer (essential) naps.

An Ancient Ritual with Modern Rewards: The Benefits of Napping

A *nap* is a short period of sleep, usually taken during the day. Napping may seem like a Mediterranean phenomenon, but one-third of American adults say that they nap.

The following sections cover some of the amazing benefits of napping.

Increasing alertness and productivity

Napping increases on-the-job alertness by 100 percent. It can increase productivity and help you improve your thinking so you can make better decisions. Napping can help to speed up your ability to perform motor tasks such as typing, operating machinery, and driving, as well as improve your accuracy on all fronts.

According to the National Sleep Foundation (NSF),

> Naps can restore alertness, enhance performance, and reduce mistakes and accidents. A study at NASA on sleepy military pilots and astronauts found that a 40-minute nap improved performance by 34 percent and alertness 100 percent. Naps can increase alertness in the period directly following the nap and may extend alertness a few hours later in the day.

Napping is also good for brain health. According to the NSF, "A nap can be a pleasant luxury, a mini-vacation. It can provide an easy way to get some relaxation and rejuvenation."

Studies revealed emergency room nurses to be much more productive and efficient after taking 25-minute naps during their shifts.

Increasing libido

Napping has been shown to increase libido, especially in women. The relationship between sleep and sexual desire and arousal is well documented. Not getting enough sleep decreases desire and arousal in women, making napping a perfect antidote. At the same time, the neurotransmitter serotonin regulates sleep, appetite, and mood and helps you to achieve a sense of satisfaction. The body consumes more serotonin during stressful situations, which is why you experience negative moods. When you nap, however, additional serotonin is released, and irritability, worry, anxiety, and depression are kept at bay.

Balancing hormones

Growth hormones and testosterone levels are reduced with lack of sleep. Both growth hormone and testosterone are powerful anabolic hormones that work together to enhance growth and body composition.

Avoiding the afternoon slumps

By reducing the amounts of mental and physical tension you feel, naps help prepare you for the rest of your day without feeling the afternoon slumps. They also help to reduce sleepiness, improve learning, and regulate emotions for the rest of the day.

Improving overall sleep time in older adults

According to research at the Weill Cornell Medical College published in the *Journal of the American Geriatrics Society*, "napping not only increases older individuals' total sleep time — without producing daytime drowsiness — but also provides measurable cognitive benefits."

Reducing the risk of a cardiovascular event

A 2019 study found that participants who took naps were 48 percent less likely to have a cardiovascular event. Taking a short nap between the hours of 1 and 3 p.m. has the most benefits.

IDEAL NAP TIMES

According to sleep specialists, the ideal nap time is 10 to 20 minutes. In the Mediterranean region, people usually punctuate the end of their meals with a cup of coffee or tea. Recently, American doctors have found that the practice of drinking a cup of coffee before taking a nap helps you to not nap for more than 30 minutes (because the caffeine begins to wake you up). If you prefer, you can just set an alarm to limit your nap time.

If you avoid naps because you worry you'll wake up feeling confused, groggy, or disoriented (known as *sleep inertia*), the key is to take a shorter nap. Ten to 20 minutes may be all you need to refresh and "reboot" your system. If you need to learn a lot of new material, longer naps of around an hour will help. During this time, the brain can transfer information from the hippocampus (where it's temporarily held) to the cortex (where it will be stored permanently).

There is evidence that different amounts of napping are beneficial to different age groups, just as different nighttime sleeping is. Johns Hopkins University researchers examined a large study of people 65 years of age and older from China and found that people who napped for 30 to 90 minutes had better word recall and were better at figure drawing than people who didn't nap or who napped for more than 90 minutes. These findings show the effects of napping on memory and cognition.

Losing weight

Sleep plays a role in weight loss, and naps can be helpful in ensuring you get enough sleep. *Metabolism* (the conversion of food to energy) is mostly affected by *muscle mass* (the weight of the muscles in your body) and hormones, but napping may be able to alter metabolism for the better. The overall health benefits that napping causes — such as better moods, higher concentration levels, and better physical health — also play their own indirect roles in helping you to lose weight because they help you to boost your metabolism. The better you feel mentally, the better food choices you'll make. The better you feel physically, the more exercise and activity you'll be able to engage in.

Many overweight people and people trying to get in shape complain of being tired. An afternoon nap can provide the energy you need to get better workouts more often. Increased, effective physical activity helps burn calories and build muscle.

Hormones play a big part in weight loss. Here are three that matter a lot:

>> **Leptin and ghrelin:** If the hunger hormones leptin and ghrelin are left unbalanced, the appetite increases and you overeat. Napping balances these hormones, reducing your appetite.

>> **Cortisol:** High amounts of the stress hormone cortisol cause inflammation, which leads to weight gain and belly fat. The stress hormone cortisol is also reduced by napping.

A study published in *Archives of Internal Medicine* found that people who are at a healthy weight get 16 minutes more sleep per day than those who are overweight. Harvard Medical School revealed that people can burn 10 percent more calories while resting in the afternoon than they do when resting in the morning.

REMEMBER

At the end of the day, diet and exercise still play the largest role in weight loss, but getting enough sleep sets the stage for diet and exercise to work.

Incorporating More Naps into Your Life

Given that memory improvement, mood enhancement, improved alertness, reduced stress and fatigue, and increased feelings of overall relaxation are all benefits of napping, you would think naps would be a national requirement. But in the United States, we're not quite there yet, so it may take some creative thinking and even stubbornness on your part, as well as a willingness to go against the grain, to successfully incorporate more naps in your daily life.

If you believe that a short nap in the afternoons could help to improve your health, not to mention your productivity, here are some easy ways to sneak them in. When the naysayers around you comment on your high productivity, good mood, or weight loss, feel free to share your secret with them!

>> **Start by avoiding serious or stressful discussions at lunch.** This will help you to relax and get a better-quality nap. A little light meditation or listening to some soothing music can help you drift to sleep if you're having difficulty.

>> **If you aren't used to sleeping in the afternoon, get yourself mentally prepared.** Turn off the lights, close the curtains, and practice deep breathing to relax.

>> **Start napping on your days off, like the weekends.** Schedule after-lunch naps on days that you don't have to work. Set aside 30 minutes of time between 1 and 3 p.m. (The shorter the nap, the less likely it is to impact your sleeping patterns.) If you work an early-day schedule, nap immediately upon coming home (before the second part of your day).

>> **Eat a meal followed by a cup of coffee before the nap.**

>> **If you work from home or don't work, schedule your appointments or online work with a half-hour break for a nap in the afternoon.** This way, you'll have enough time to doze off and wake back up again.

>> **Meditate.** Closing your eyes to meditate — even if it's just for 5 minutes after a lunch at the office — can relax the mind and help you to sleep better in the evening.

TIP

If an afternoon nap is absolutely out of the question due to your schedule, getting extra sleep at night will also be beneficial.

Sometimes napping just may not work out for you. If you frequently nap for a long time and you have trouble sleeping at night, or if it's too late in the evening when you have time to nap, you may want to save the experience for when you're free to doze off earlier in the day.

TIP

Want to make the most of your nap? Here are a few easy techniques to incorporate:

>> **Cover yourself with a blanket.** The body loses some of its heat when it's at rest, and it's common to feel a bit cold upon waking.

>> **Keep your head raised during a nap — don't lay down totally flat.** The physiological benefits of napping have been shown to be increased when people keep their heads raised high during naps.

» **Try to nap in a cool space with the lights dimmed.** No need for total darkness — that will only confuse your body into thinking it's nighttime.

» **Minimize unwanted sound while napping.** Certain sounds, such as nature or other things that you have positive feelings toward, can help you, but noises you find annoying will only distract.

» **Change your clothes if possible.** If you aren't wearing comfortable clothes, slipping into something more comfortable will help you to fall asleep more easily.

» **If you simply can't fall asleep, use the time to stretch out and clear your thoughts.** Try meditation or deep breathing to help you feel better. Taking a few moments for yourself will help you feel better in both the short and long term.

3

Adopting Healthful Cultural Attitudes

IN THIS PART . . .

Get easy-to-use references, practical tools, and checklists to live your best Mediterranean life daily.

Use food and the pleasures of eating as a metaphor for life.

Chapter **10**

Living Mediterranean-Style Daily

Regardless of which Mediterranean country you spend time in, you'll be able to see that daily life is a colorful mosaic of millennia-old cultural traditions, wisdom, and ingenuity, combined with modern conveniences and an ancient zest for life. Whether you're in Algeria or Crete or Syria, the ways of life are woven so deeply into the fabric of everyday life, that most people from the region take their health-boosting customs for granted — until they travel abroad to countries that don't practice them.

In this chapter, I explain many of the daily living traditions that often get overlooked in discussions about the Mediterranean lifestyle. I also give you a tour of all the countries in the region so you can discover the easiest and best ways to reap the rewards of Mediterranean living.

The ABCs of the Mediterranean Lifestyle

As a Mediterranean Lifestyle Ambassador, I've come up with a lexicon to help people associate certain activities with the Mediterranean lifestyle, underline their importance, and serve as a reminder to do these activities as often as possible:

Agriculture	Sustainable traditions yield better food.
Bread and **B**eauty	Bread is the backbone of the diet and culinary culture. Beauty is a concept valued by everyone in each area of daily life.
Community and **C**ulture	Acting, thinking, and eating for the benefit of the community and in a way that promotes cultural traditions.
D (the vitamin)	The sun provides a lot of vitamin D naturally.
Extra-virgin olive oil	Extra-virgin olive oil is the go-to cooking fat, flavor enhancer, and traditional medicinal.
Fresh air	Fresh air is prized for its health benefits.
Gardening	Most people in the Mediterranean enjoy gardening, whether on a balcony, on a rooftop, on a windowsill, or in a garden.
Home cooking	Home cooking is valued and prized for its important role in our overall health and in maintaining a culture's customs.
Inclusion	"The more the merrier" is usually the rule of thumb, and togetherness is preferred to being alone.
Joy	Joy is the ultimate daily goal and the reason for adopting as many pleasurable activities as possible.
Kin	Family matters most throughout the Mediterranean.
Laughter	Laughter is a natural remedy used to lift the spirits as often as possible.
Music	Music is an important part of every Mediterranean culture and enjoyed daily, not just on special occasions.
Nature	Nature is beloved, and people go the extra mile to preserve their communities' environments.
Outdoors	In the Mediterranean, people spend as much time outdoors or with a view of the outdoors as possible.
Purpose, **P**roduce, and **P**lants	A reason for living can be personal or collective, but knowing and acting on your purpose is essential for happiness to most people in the region. Fresh fruits and vegetables make up the bulk of the diet. Cultivate as many plants as possible — both for personal gratification and for the environment.

Quality	Quality is always chosen over quantity.
Rest and **R**elaxation	Rest and relaxation are important daily practices.
Sunlight	Sunlight leads to a sunny disposition and optimism. Seasonal affective disorder is not an issue in the Mediterranean region because people intentionally plan ways to incorporate more sun into their days, even in the winter months.
Traditions	Many people in the Mediterranean are working diligently to promote traditions from previous generations for the future as a means of preserving culture, identity, and more.
Unity	In the Mediterranean, a premium is placed on doing things together. This tradition has deep roots in maintaining peace between tribes and within communities. People work diligently to create common ground among those who have differing viewpoints instead of avoiding sensitive topics.
Value	Price is not the only way to measure the worth of an activity or object. Value in the Mediterranean region is assigned to things that enhance life, health, the environment, and the community, and people are willing to pay more money for those things.
Water	In addition to hydrotherapy, the healing effects of water and drinking enough from clean sources — often mineral springs — are promoted.
Xenia	*Xenia* is the Ancient Greek concept of hospitality, which is at the core of every Mediterranean culture. Locals strive to be good hosts in the way that other cultures may strive to win an award or get a promotion. The role of a host is taken very seriously, and to be a good host speaks to a person's character.
Young at heart	In an area that is home to many centenarians and highly functioning elderly people, keeping a youthful attitude is important. Letting go of concerns easily and fostering a childlike wonder for life are key factors.
Zeal	My Greek friends and I call this the "opa!" factor for the Greek exclamation that connotes a zest for life. A deep appreciation for life itself and a desire to live it to the fullest are commonplace in the region.

Getting a Mediterranean Lifestyle Checklist

People who've lived or grown up in the Mediterranean region don't need a check-list to remind them of healthful and pleasurable activities to participate in. In fact, checklists themselves go a bit against the grain of the free-flowing Mediterranean lifestyle. That said, checklists are a great way for beginners to get familiar with habits that are new to them. You can copy or cut out the checklist and place it on a refrigerator or office wall so you remember which activities really matter in terms of well-being. When you're fluent in these practices, keeping a list around is no longer necessary, and the quality of your life will improve greatly.

Here's my Mediterranean lifestyle checklist:

- ❑ **Grow and use fresh herbs in your home or garden.** You can use a simple windowsill or a cart placed in front of a window to grow healthful herbs — you don't need a big yard.

- ❑ **Cook a meal for yourself and/or your family.** Take pleasure in making more of your meals at home and sharing them with others for the mental and physical payoff.

- ❑ **Decide who to eat with before deciding what to eat.** Eating communally is the backbone of the Mediterranean lifestyle — the more, the merrier!

- ❑ **Base each meal around produce.** Decide which fresh, local vegetables you love, and make them the base of your meals.

- ❑ **Buy organic groceries when possible.** Better-quality food leads to better health.

- ❑ **Eat with others as often as possible.** Look for creative ways to include other people in your mealtimes — even if it means going outside of familial bonds and using unconventional methods such as FaceTime and Skype to do so.

- ❑ **Engage in physical activity that you enjoy.** Doing what you love is as good for the psyche as physical exercise is for the body. Pick some activities you really enjoy, and you'll get total body benefits at the same time. If you add nature into the mix, you'll be getting three benefits at once!

- ❑ **Participate in a hobby or activity that you enjoy.** This activity adds meaning and pleasure in your life while contributing to your purpose and lowering stress.

- ❑ **Visit a farm.** Seeing where your food comes from helps you to be more in tune with what's seasonal and local. Often you can pick your own ingredients, which means more exercise and fresh air!

- ❑ **Attend a food festival.** Food festivals are a great way to celebrate local ingredients, learn new recipes, and support the community while spending time outdoors.

- ❑ **Learn a new recipe.** This activity provides a sense of accomplishment while increasing your cooking skills and confidence.

- ❏ **Teach someone a new recipe.** Passing along knowledge is mentally satisfying and helps to boost relationships and camaraderie.

- ❏ **Bring or make a healthy lunch on workdays.** You'll enjoy nutritionally sound meals and save money.

- ❏ **Use good-quality extra-virgin olive oil as your main cooking fat.** This healthful fat provides powerful antioxidants and omega-3 fatty acids, which work to coax additional nutrients out of healthful foods and have anti-inflammatory properties that help keep many diseases at bay.

- ❏ **Take a walk outdoors after a meal.** Walking after a meal improves digestion and increases your exposure to nature and the outdoors.

- ❏ **Spend time gardening or with potted plants.** A recent study revealed that gardening was linked to greater happiness along with eating out, biking, walking, and recreational activities.

- ❏ **Shop at a farmers market when possible.** You'll be able to form relationships with local food providers, get access to the best foods available, and be part of your community.

- ❏ **Enjoy healthful foods as the base of each meal.** Make sure that your meals are based on healthful ingredients such as leafy greens, cruciferous vegetables, beans, legumes, whole grains, fish and seafood, and dairy, with good-quality meat eaten sparingly.

- ❏ **Use aromatics to flavor food.** Instead of adding more salt, butter, and cream to recipes to make your food taste better, opt for good-quality spices, handfuls of chopped fresh herbs, garlic, onions, and shallots to produce more taste without the calories and fat.

- ❏ **Create meat-free meals when possible.** Many Americans base their meals around meat. Swapping the meat out for fish, chicken, dairy, or plant-based protein (such as legumes and soy), even a few times a week, will make a difference.

- ❏ **Choose fruit for dessert.** On regular days, instead of finishing a meal with a fat- and calorie-laden dessert, grab a piece of fresh fruit instead. You'll get a dose of sweetness along with vitamins and minerals. Save the super-sweet treats for special occasions or once a week.

- ❏ **Start or maintain a healthful eating ritual with friends or family.** If you can, start a tradition of eating at least one meal a day with friends, family, colleagues, or others who value the benefits of communal eating.

- ❏ **Add an additional serving of fish to your weekly diet.** Just one additional serving per week can reduce your risk of heart disease by 49 percent while providing healthful fats and brainpower-boosting nutrients.

- ❑ **Aim for 5 to 12 servings of fresh fruits and vegetables daily.** Eating lots of leafy green vegetables along with the "rainbow" of colors in produce every day is an easy way to fill up on fiber while ensuring that you're getting a wide range of nutrients.

- ❑ **Add leafy green vegetables to your lunch and dinner menus.** Artichokes, asparagus, avocado, broccoli, Brussels sprouts, cabbage, celery, chicory, collard greens, dandelion greens, kale, kiwi, lettuce, purslane, spinach, Swiss chard, and zucchini are examples of nutrient-dense produce. Be sure to add at least one of them to every meal.

- ❑ **Stock a pantry with healthful, Mediterranean options.** Turn to Chapter 14 for more information.

- ❑ **Create a week's worth of Mediterranean menus for each meal before making a shopping list.** Turn to Chapter 13 for more on this subject.

- ❑ **Bring healthful snacks, such as fruit and nuts, with you when you leave home.** This will stave off hunger longer and ensure that you aren't satisfying your hunger with something unhealthy.

- ❑ **Listen to beautiful music whenever possible.** Music will help boost your mood, energy, and concentration. Grapes grow better and are more resistant to disease when classical music is played in vineyards, so imagine what it can do for your body!

- ❑ **Beautify your space with objects that are meaningful to you.** We all have our own definitions of beauty and what's meaningful to us. The more of those elements that you can add to your work and home space, the better.

- ❑ **Choose quality over quantity.** No matter the topic, quality always beats out quantity in the Mediterranean region. Older cultures appreciate things that last and are willing to have less variety in order to have something that will stand the test of time.

- ❑ **Talk with a close confidante.** Having someone to confide in is integral to mental health.

- ❑ **Get a minimum of 30 minutes of fresh air per day.** Mental health professionals claim that fresh air is more beneficial to our moods than antipsychotic drugs are.

- ❑ **Laugh as often as possible.** Lowering stress and increasing happiness is great for healing and preventing illness.

- ❑ **Make time for rest and relaxation.** Rest and relaxation are a daily, not a once-a-year, practice in the Mediterranean region.

- ❑ **Look on the bright side of situations that are bothersome in your life.** Making the best out of whatever life deals you is an art form in the Mediterranean.

❑ **Spend time in nature, preferably by water and/or green trees.** The "green effect" and the "blue effect" of spending just 10 minutes a day looking at trees or water have emotional benefits.

❑ **Practice gratitude for blessings large and small as often as possible.** "If you say only one prayer, make it thank you" is a popular philosophy in the region, and this attitude helps attract more of the things we love.

❑ **Live your purpose in every way possible.** This will add meaning to your days and make living worthwhile.

❑ **Eat your larger meal at lunchtime.** In the middle of the day, you still have time to burn off more calories, and it will help you to maintain a healthier weight and sleep better.

❑ **Take a 10- to 20-minute nap.** Naps help productivity, focus, weight management, stress reduction, and much more.

❑ **Aim for 6 to 8 hours of sleep every night.** Getting enough sleep promotes better overall body functions, such as blood sugar management, hormonal functions, and brain performance.

❑ **Create a DIY project.** Having a project promotes a sense of accomplishment and purpose.

❑ **Participate in a cultural activity (for example, theater, opera, or a sporting event) with loved ones.** Socialization increases the level of oxytocin (known as the "love hormone").

❑ **Host guests for a meal, coffee, or tea.** Even a small gesture goes a long way toward promoting feelings of camaraderie and community.

❑ **Organize your day around your meals as much as possible.** This ensures eating the right foods at the right times while promoting a sense of security and safety.

❑ **Drink herbal teas in the evening before bed and throughout the day.** The nutritional benefits of herbs can help in achieving our various health goals and are healthful, caffeine-free rituals.

❑ **Eat 1 serving of beans or legumes per day.** Most Americans fall short in this category, but these foods are an important part of the Mediterranean diet.

❑ **Spend some time in the sun.** Getting more vitamin D helps immunity, while sun exposure increases serotonin (a mood stabilizer).

❑ **Contribute to charity or volunteer your time.** In addition to helping the community, volunteering helps to increase oxytocin.

❑ **Peruse philosophy books.** Philosophy helps us to understand ourselves, the world we live in, and how we relate to it.

❑ **Practice ethical and/or spiritual traditions that are symbolic to you.** These traditions add meaning, ritual, and routine to life, while offering support mechanisms during times of adversity.

❑ **Cook with as many local ingredients as possible.** Our bodies crave the nutrients found in produce that's in season in the regions we live in. In addition to saving money and supporting the environment, eating locally is better for your health.

❑ **Engage in community efforts as often as possible.** Strong community relationships provide psychological security and advantages.

❑ **Foster fabulous friendships.** Having a few trustworthy friends and confidents is important for mental well-being.

❑ **Strive for authenticity in your relationships.** Being genuine and sincere is the best way to foster healthy relationships.

An Overview of Mediterranean Cultures

Nowadays, dozens of countries border the Mediterranean Sea. After millennia of converging cultural influences, many common customs and traditions prevail, while each nation and geographic location within those nations have their own distinguishing features. Entire books could be written about each country, island, or state in the region, but this list serves as a simple way to note the vast range of inspiration that is ripe for the picking in these alluring lands.

Albania

Albanian culture is created from a blend of the indigenous Illyrians in antiquity and has also been influenced by the Ancient Greeks, Romans, Byzantines, and Ottomans. Today religious equality is an important value in the country, which has significant Christian and Muslim populations. The Albanian language is the official language, and two dialects (Tosk and Gheg) are spoken there. Many Albanians also learn to speak English, French, German, Greek, and Italian due to the large *diaspora*. Between the 14th and 18th centuries, many Albanians fled their homeland to settle in other European countries. In Southern Italy, there is a community of Albanians known as Arbëreshë, who descended from the Tosk culture and maintain their language and culture while living in Italy. Albanians live in Greece and other Mediterranean cultures as well.

Algeria

Located in North Africa, the official languages of Algeria are Arabic and Tamazight, a dialect of the indigenous people often referred to as Berber in the history books. The politically correct term *Amazigh* became the official language alongside Arabic in 2016. After French colonization, the French language was widely used in government and education, even though it isn't an official language. Kabyle, the most spoken indigenous language in the country, is taught by millions of Algerians in other regions, and other dialects are spoken as well. Phoenicians and Romans coexisted with the indigenous people of Algeria for centuries. The Amazigh people were Christianized during the Roman Empire. Berbers became Islamized after the Muslim conquest of the region under the Umayyad Caliphate from Syria.

Bosnia and Herzegovina

The Bosnian, Serbian, and Croatian languages are all spoken in the land that is commonly referred to as Bosnia. Located in South and Southeast Europe, within the Balkans, Bosnia and Herzegovina has had permanent human settlement since the Neolithic Age, when it was inhabited by the Butmir, Kakanj, and Vučedol peoples. It was then populated by several Illyrian and Celtic civilizations. After the 14th century, it was annexed into the Ottoman Empire, under whose rule it remained until the late 19th century. The Ottomans brought Islam to the region and left a permanent mark on the local culture, which was annexed into the Austro-Hungarian Empire and later became a part of Yugoslavia, until it became independent in 1995.

Croatia

Croatia's culture is a mix of earlier Greek, Roman, and Bronze Age influences, combined with Serbian, Italian, and Catholic elements. Expressed in early times in music, dance, art, and Catholicism's magnificent architecture, its visual elements were also influenced by the Venetian Renaissance period. The Roman, Ottoman, and Austrian-Hungarian empires all left their mark on this small yet culturally rich country. Standard Croatian is the official language of the nation, as well as one of the official languages of Bosnia-Herzegovina. It's also official in the regions of Burgenland (Austria), Molise (Italy), and Vojvodina (Serbia).

Cyprus

The island of Cyprus is culturally divided into the Turkish northern part (where Turkish is spoken and many names have been changed to Turkish) and the southern Greek part (where the Greek language is still spoken). The town of Paphos, the legendary birthplace of Aphrodite, is home to a 12th century BCE temple constructed in her honor. The island also boasts United Nations Educational, Scientific, and Cultural Organization (UNESCO) World Heritage sites, which boast its Byzantine and Neolithic origins. Levantine, Anatolian, and Greek influences are present in everything from the cuisine of the island to its folklore and handicrafts.

Egypt

Ever since the days of the Ancient Egyptian Empire, the "Mother of the World" has been connecting East, West, North, and South in the Mediterranean region. Much of the earliest cross-cultural trade in the Mediterranean basin started in Egypt. The official language spoken is Arabic, and Egypt has its own dialect that is understood throughout the Arab world due to the Egyptian film and music industry, which is widely followed in all Arabic-speaking countries. Here, Nubian, Pharaonic, Jewish, Roman, Greek, Arab, Ottoman, French, and English influences combined to create a culture like no other. Egypt's population today is predominately Sunni Muslim, with a large Coptic Christian minority. Egypt has the second-largest economy in Africa.

France

Some people don't consider France to be part of the Mediterranean, but its southernmost region of Provence is as quintessentially Mediterranean as any other place in the region. Provence takes its name from the Latin *Provincia Romana*, from Roman times; it also has Greek and Phoenician roots. Although French is the official language, the Provençal dialect actually is very similar to the dialect spoken in the Italian Riviera because, prior to the 19th century, they were ruled by the same kingdom. The two areas also share many similar foods and entertainment styles. Archeologists have also found Phoenician trading ships in the Mediterranean Sea just off the coast of France, which reveals evidence of the trading that took place from modern-day Lebanon all the way to France.

Greece

What we now consider to be the Mediterranean diet was originally known as the Greek diet, and most of its criteria came from the island of Crete. Modern Greek is the official language of Greece, and its inhabitants practice the Greek Orthodox faith, which has had a major role in developing dietary trends. Ancient Greek philosophers such as Pythagoras and Epicurus also spoke extensively about nutrition, as did Hippocrates, the father of modern medicine. The first known western cookbook author, Archestratus, wrote his cookbook in the 4th century BCE on the island of Sicily, which was then part of Magna Graecia. The Greeks also colonized parts of Provence, as well as the coastline of all of Southern Europe, the Levant, and parts of North Africa in ancient times. The Greek culture has been influenced not only by its own ancient civilizations, but also by Central Asian, Anatolian, Egyptian, Italian, French, and Ottoman influences as well.

Israel

Home to several sacred sites in Jerusalem, Israel is significant to Jews, Christians, and Muslims as the biblical Holy Land. The historic city's Temple Mount complex includes the Dome of the Rock (which is sacred to Muslims), the historic Western Wall (which is sacred to Jews), the Al-Aqsa Mosque (which is sacred to Muslims), and the Church of the Holy Sepulcher (which is sacred to Christians). Israel defines itself as a Jewish and democratic state and the nation-state of the Jewish people. Inhabited by Canaanite tribes since the Bronze Age, Ancient Judah was later conquered by the Babylonian, Persian, Hellenistic, Byzantine, Arab, and Ottoman empires, each of which had control of Israel over various points in time. Home to the seven food species listed in the Old Testament (Deuteronomy 8:8) —wheat, barley, grape, fig, pomegranates, olive (oil), and date (honey) — the indigenous foods of The Holy Land perfectly exemplify the Mediterranean diet. Nowadays, the country's religious makeup is predominately Jewish, with a large Muslim and small Christian and Druze minorities. Hebrew is the official language of Israel, and Arabic is widely spoken as well. Israeli cuisine is largely based on indigenous Palestinian dishes that have been made there for millennia, along with dishes from the Jewish diaspora and Jewish immigrants to Israel from Eastern Europe, North Africa, Ethiopia, Yemen, Iraq, the Soviet Union, and beyond.

Italy

The Mediterranean diet is deeply rooted in the Cilento area, where American researcher Dr. Ansel Keyes lived. Nicotera in Calabria was another rural area studied for its diet in the famous Seven Countries Study. The Italian island of Sardinia boasts the world's largest number of centenarians and is a Blue Zone (see Chapter 4). Italy's citizens are often voted the healthiest people in Europe for their diet and lifestyle. Italian is the official language of Italy, but prior to unification in the mid 19th century, each of Italy's now 20 regions was home to several different dialects. Many culinary and daily living terms are referred to by locals in dialect today, even though the language is standardized. Most Italians are of the Roman Catholic faith, which along with the pagan faiths of the indigenous tribes contributed to many of the cultural connections of the lifestyle. Italian food is the most popular food in the United States and around the world.

WARNING

There is a lot of imitation and counterfeit "Italian" food on the market that bears no nutritional or traditional resemblance to the real deal. These unhealthful imitation dishes ruin the reputation of Italian food and have nothing to do with the Mediterranean diet. If you're seeking the heath-boosting benefits of authentic Italian cuisine, seek out genuine Italian food made with the freshest produce, beans, legumes, grains, seafood, and dairy.

Lebanon

Often called the "Switzerland of the East" or the "Paris of the East" because of its natural beauty and gorgeous mountain ranges and the cosmopolitan nature of Beirut. Lebanon is known for its cuisine and culture, both of which have been popularized around the world thanks to its large diaspora. (There are more Lebanese people living abroad than in the country itself.) It's bordered by Syria to the north and east and Israel to the south, while Cyprus lies just west of it across the Mediterranean Sea. Arabic is the official language, and the Lebanese have their own dialect of Arabic as well. Today Lebanon is also known for its fashion designers. Civilization began here 7,000 years ago, and the land was home to the Phoenicians, a seafaring culture that flourished for almost 3,000 years (from about 3200 to 539 BCE) and set up trading centers all the way from Lebanon to France. In 64 BCE, the Roman Empire conquered the region and introduced Christianity. The Maronites, the primary Eastern Catholic group in Lebanon, and the Druze also established themselves in Mount Lebanon. Later, Arab rule took over and the country was populated by the Ottomans from the 16th century to the 20th century, when Lebanon fell into the hands of the French. Because of the large number of Lebanese people living abroad, most Arabic food available in the Americas is Lebanese.

Libya

Libya is a North African country nestled between Algeria, Tunisia, Chad, Niger, and Egypt and bordered by the Mediterranean Sea. Indigenous tribes were there in the Bronze Age. They were followed by the Ancient Egyptians, Greeks, Phoenicians, Carthaginians, Persians, and Romans, all of whom laid claim to the land prior to the Arab conquests. Libya is the 4th-largest country in Africa and the 16th-largest country in the world, with seven million inhabitants who speak Arabic. From 1934 to 1947, Libya was an Italian colony. Libyans are predominantly considered Arabs; 96 percent are Sunni Muslims who live along the Mediterranean coastline.

Malta

Independent since 1964, the island of Malta, nestled between Sicily and North Africa in the Mediterranean Sea, has a history going back more than 7,000 years. The official Maltese language was Italian until 1934, but the names of numbers were pronounced in Arabic. Today the official language is Maltese, which is a Sicilian Arabic that was spoken when Sicily was considered an emirate. English is the official second language and many people still speak Italian. There you'll witness some of the oldest freestanding temples in the world. The republic also hosted the Phoenicians, Romans, Greeks, Carthaginians, Arabs, Knights of St. John, Napoleon, and the British Empire.

Monaco

The Principality of Monaco is the second-smallest sovereign state in the world after Vatican City. Located on the French Riviera close to the Italian region of Liguria, Monaco was ruled by the House of Grimaldi, founded by rulers in Genoa, Italy, until the mid-19th century. Bordered by France to the north, east, and west, and the Mediterranean Sea to the south, the principality has approximately 38,000 residents, The official language is French, although Monegasque (a dialect of Ligurian), Italian, and English are spoken and understood by many there. Prince Albert II is head of state, and the defense of the principality is under the responsibility of the French.

Montenegro

Located on the Adriatic Sea in the Balkans, Montenegro (which means "Black Mountain") is a founding member of the Union of the Mediterranean and is in the process of becoming a member of the European Union. The Venetian Republic, Venetian Albania, the Ottoman Empire, Yugoslavia, Serbia, and Bosnia have all played a role in the cultural makeup of the country. The languages it uses are Serbian, Albanian, Bosnian, and Croatian. It terms of ethnicity, the country is made up of 45.0 percent Montenegrins, 28.7 percent Serbs, 8.6 percent Bosnians, 4.9 percent Albanians, and 12.7% other. The majority of the population is Christian, with 72 percent practicing Eastern Orthodoxy and 19 percent practicing Islam.

Morocco

The Arabic name for Morocco is *Maghreb* (which means "where the sun sets"), because it was the westernmost region of the Islamic Empire. The Arabic word for sunset is, in fact, *el Maghreb,* which is the same name for the kingdom. Arabic, French, and a standard Moroccan version of the indigenous languages of the

Amazigh, known as Tamazight, are the official languages of the nation, whose motto is "God, Homeland, King," a slogan that you will see over and over again on trips there. Located in Northwestern Africa, the country is made up of approximately 99 percent Sunni Muslims whose manner of worship incorporates a significant amount of Sufism. The kingdom was also home to a large Jewish population that was indigenous to Morocco and was a safe haven to Jews fleeing persecution during the Spanish Inquisition. Ruled by King Mohammed VI, Morocco is home to 37,112,080 people, as of the 2020 census. The first Moroccan state was founded by Idris I in 788 CE, and in addition to its indigenous Amazigh roots, the nation has hosted Romans, Greeks, several Muslim dynasties, Portugal, France, and Spain. It's worth noting that Morocco is the only North African nation that escaped Ottoman occupation and is now the fifth-largest economy in Africa.

Slovenia

The Republic of Slovenia is located in Central Europe and is bordered by Italy, Austria, Hungary, and Croatia. It's a predominately Catholic country with an Eastern Orthodox minority population. The history of this highly developed nation begins in prehistory and includes Roman and Slavic influences, as well as Croatian, Serbian, Slovenian, Yugoslavian, and more. Ethnically speaking, the majority of the country's population consists of Slovenes, with a large Serb minority. Slovene is the official language. Culturally speaking, the country has been influenced by Slavic, German, and Latin languages and cultures. Slovenia's high-income economy ranks it very high on the Human Development Index, which is a marker of life expectancy, education, and per capita income indicators.

Spain

The Kingdom of Spain is consistently associated with the Mediterranean diet and lifestyle in the United States. In 2021, Money.co.uk named Spain the world's healthiest country based on life expectancy, the affordability of a healthy lifestyle, air quality, and obesity rates. By following Mediterranean diet and lifestyle doctrines, Spanish people suffer from fewer diseases compared to the rest of the world. The official language is Spanish, and 84.8 percent of the population are Spaniards, with a large percentage Roman Catholics. Ruled by King Felipe VI, Spain has a long history with influences from across the Mediterranean. Situated on the Iberian Peninsula, its territory also includes two archipelagos: the Canary Islands off the coast of North Africa, and the Balearic Islands in the Mediterranean Sea. Bordered by the Mediterranean Sea, Portugal, and France, Spain is also connected to Morocco. The fourth most populated country in the European Union has been inhabited for 42,000 years. Phoenicians, Greeks, Celts, Carthaginians, Basques, and Romans all had a presence in Ancient Iberia.

Syria

The oldest alphabet, oldest song, and oldest painting in the world were all discovered in what is now Syria. Recently, the Oriental Institute in Chicago held a musical performance of a modern interpretation of "The Prayer of Infertility," which was the world's first known song. Syria is home to 22 different religious and ethnic sects. The capital city, Damascus, is now the cultural capital of the Arab world. Syria is also home to a monastery that has become an important pilgrimage site for Christians, one of the oldest and largest mosques in the world, and synagogues. Pagan gods, Christian saints, revered Jewish religious figures, and many Muslim prophets and caliphs once walked on the ancient crossroads in Damascus, the world's oldest continuously inhabited city. The official language of Syria is Arabic, and the country is located in Western Asia. A country of fertile plains, high mountains, and deserts, it borders Lebanon, the Mediterranean Sea, Turkey, Iraq, Jordan, and Israel. Syrian Arabs, Kurds, Turkmens, Assyrians, Armenians, Circassians, Mandaeans, and Greeks are all part of the cultural makeup of the country. Religious groups include a majority of Sunni Muslims, along with Christians, Alawites, Druze, and several other minorities. Including everything from the Babylonian and Assyrian empires, the deep and rich history of Syria is so varied that to name each group that contributed to its heritage would make too long a list. Aleppo was the third-largest city in the Ottoman Empire, after Constantinople and Cairo. Their years of converging cultures left a deep imprint on everything from cuisine to music and literature. The first Muslim Caliphate, the Umayyads, were based in Damascus; they introduced city dwelling, spread Islam throughout the Mediterranean region, and later ruled Spain.

Tunisia

The Republic of Tunisia is the northernmost country in Africa. It's located just across the Mediterranean Sea from Italy and is bordered by Algeria, Libya, and the Mediterranean. Tunisia has a population of only 11 million people, much less than the population of the cities of Cairo and Istanbul alone. Tunisia was originally inhabited by the indigenous Amazigh people. Then the Phoenicians inhabited the area. Finally, Carthage emerged as the most powerful force in Tunisia in the 7th century BCE. A major mercantile empire and a military rival of the Roman Republic, Carthage was defeated in 146 BCE by the Romans, who occupied Tunisia for most of the next 800 years, introducing Christianity and leaving architectural landmarks. Muslims conquered all of Tunisia by 697 CE, bringing Islam and Arab culture to the local inhabitants. Several different Muslim caliphates ruled the nation and introduced their own influences. In the tenth century, two separate groups based in modern-day Tunisia were very influential in the Mediterranean region.

Tunisia's influence expands far beyond the borders of the small Mediterranean country. Both the Aghlabids and Fatimids claimed rule in Sicily during that period, and their presence forever changed the Italian (as well as that of other places) culinary and cultural landscape. The Aghlabids introduced things such as lemons, oranges, the tradition of making gelato, mulberries, eggplant, and many other ingredients to Italy. The Fatimids (who took their name from the Prophet Mohammed's daughter) were responsible for naming the city of Palermo, and they claimed it 50 years before they claimed Cairo. They promoted cross-religious holiday celebrations. During their rule, Jews, Christians, and Muslims celebrated together. As a result, many of the foods that they promoted, such as the art of sesame candy and nougat making, became associated with religious celebrations in all three faiths. These caliphates linked Tunis to Morocco, Southern Spain, Sicily, all of North Africa, Egypt, and the Muslim Holy Cities in Saudi Arabia. Later the Ottoman Empire established control in 1574, and remained in power for 300 years, until the French conquered Tunisia in 1881. Tunisia gained independence in 1957, and it's now the smallest nation in North Africa. Tunisia's cosmopolitan culture reflects both its maritime roots and the combination of various ethnic influences that have inhabited it.

Turkey

The Republic of Turkey spans Western Asia and Southeast Europe. It's bordered by Greece, Bulgaria, the Black Sea, Georgia, Armenia, Azerbaijan, Iran, Iraq, Syria, the Mediterranean Sea, and the Aegean Sea. Istanbul is the largest city in Turkey. For many centuries, Istanbul was a sister city of Venice and Cairo. The spice trade flourished between these three urban centers, building their power and wealth.

One of the world's earliest permanently settled areas, Turkey hosts important Neolithic sites and peoples, such as the Hattian and Anatolian peoples. Greeks, Byzantines, Seljuks, Mongols, Ottomans, and many others also ruled the powerful and strategically located land. In 1923, Turkey became a secular, unitary and parliamentary republic. A newly industrialized country, Turkey is a regional power in the Middle East and is now the 20th-largest growth-leading economy in the world.

Turkey also boasted many opulent times in history. During the reign of the Ottoman Empire, for example, an authentic artisan Turkish rug was worth more money than Michelangelo's *David*. Turkish goods were so coveted that many merchants attempted to make counterfeit products with calligraphy, which was created to fool consumers in Europe who were unable to read the then-used Arabic script. Nowadays Turkish is the official language of Turkey, and Roman script is used. Just as its arts were prized, so was its cuisine. Topkapi Palace in Istanbul used to employ 1,000 chefs at a time. Each chef had 100 understudies and was only allowed to make one type of food, such as soups, dough, kebabs, or sweets. This way, if a cook passed away, the assistants would've already learned the recipe and could take over. For this reason, we have excellent records of Ottoman recipes from this period. Chefs would travel from all over the globe to learn from those palace cooks, yet many dishes were not successfully re-created at home. It is said, for example, that French puff pastry was invented after a botched attempt at paper-thin *yufka* (Turkish phyllo) dough. The Ottomans also introduced many foods via the New World and Far East to the Mediterranean, which is why Italians call cornmeal "Turkish grain." Turkish coffee was never grown in Turkey but was marketed and distributed by the Ottomans. Modern-day Turkey is a kaleidoscope of East-meets-West tradition, ingenuity, and style.

Chapter **11**

Seeing Food as a Metaphor for Life

The Mediterranean region is not the only place where people see food as a metaphor for life — in fact, most ancient cultures do. After all, in ancient times, food was a form of currency. Ancient Egypt, for example, was the chief exporter of lentils, which were once worth their weight in gold and used as a valuable commodity. Many medieval cities were built on the spice trade. In other words, food not only kept people alive (because it provided nutrients) but also was the basis of most ancient commodities.

Fast-forward to modern times, and you see that eating a healthful diet is still the best and most direct way to take charge of your health. Agriculture and the food industry are still essential for the survival of our species. Cooking, eating, sharing, giving, and even talking about food still inspire a level of joy and intimacy in the hearts of people worldwide.

In this chapter, you take a step back in time and see how simple shifts in thinking can improve your overall health.

Getting to Cook versus Having to Cook

Today, cooking is seen as a chore in many parts of the modern world. I often hear comments like; "Let's go out so you don't *have* to cook." Interestingly, I've never heard that sentence uttered in the Mediterranean.

Every time I hear those words, I have the same response: First, I cringe, and then I remind the person that cooking for them would be a great *joy* for me. Usually, they respond with, "Yes, but you don't *have* to for once. Why not just relax?" Then I explain that cooking *is* relaxing for me — that's why I chose it as a career — but it always falls on deaf ears. Truth be told, I feel most alive when I'm cooking, baking, and sharing food with my loved ones, so what may look like a labor of love to them (emphasis on *labor*) is just me aligning with my purpose in life.

The same thing is true for most people, especially women, in the Mediterranean region. They grew up assigning so much importance to the notion of being good hosts that they can't wait to show off their desire to take care of their guests. Of course, there are exceptions to the rule: Not everyone in Egypt, France, or Italy, for example, loves to cook. So many people do, however, that someone else in the family or their neighbors will pick up the slack, and they'll be able to enjoy delicious, high-quality, homemade food (and company!) on a regular basis.

EATING OUT: WHEN AND WHY

I love restaurants of all sorts, and I would never want to shame anyone who frequents them. It is, however, more healthy — and more Mediterranean! — to frequent restaurants for the right reasons, such as wanting to enjoy that particular restaurant's food, trying something new, enjoying the environment or the company, or savoring dishes that you normally wouldn't eat at home. Those are all great reasons to eat out!

Eating out becomes problematic, however, when it's the norm and when you've been disconnected from the joy of cooking. It becomes an issue when you think you can only enjoy a meal, or that a meal is only worthy, if someone else cooks it for you. Anytime you dread a task that you're required to do or need to do often, you set yourself up for suffering. People in the Mediterranean region, in large part, value *every* meal they eat, not just restaurant meals. They value themselves, their guests, their neighbors, their community, and their environment, as well as the crops that Mother Nature blesses their land with.

HOW COOKING FELL OUT OF FAVOR

In the United States, there was a great deal of propaganda during and after World War II that encouraged educated, wise, modern, working women (many of whom were filling in for soldiers away at war) to not "waste their time" in the kitchen. This type of mentality led to the increased usage of boxed cake mixes, industrially prepared bread with chemically based ingredients (to create a long shelf life), preservative-laden packaged foods for supermarket shelves, TV dinners, and of course, all kinds of canned goods that were needed for stocking bomb shelters with.

Many women went "back home" after the soldiers came back from the war and started working at their old jobs again. Even though women had *time* to cook, manufacturers still wanted to sell those packaged goods, and appealing to the American woman's intellect was just the way. Advertisements and marketing campaigns that portrayed women who spent too long in the kitchen as uneducated, inefficient (because they wasted time), and out of fashion bombarded the popular culture. Little by little, all those packaged goods replaced homemade ones, and two generations later one out of two American adults have diabetes or pre-diabetes. In addition, there is a widely held belief that cooking is a chore for the home cook, but an art for someone who cooks in a fancy restaurant, and most people are very far removed from the production and preparation of their own food.

Finding inspiration

The first step to enjoying cooking is gratitude and the recognition that you want to create wonderful meals for yourselves and your loved ones. In the Mediterranean region, the love of food is so celebrated because it's something that everyone can appreciate. We all have to eat to survive. But when we eat to *thrive*, mealtimes really take on a whole new meaning.

We all experience stress, and at various times in our lives, we face struggles that we have no idea how to surpass — until one day we miraculously do. Cooking — and enjoying yourself in the process — gives you an opportunity to take back the reins of your daily life and create something you love. Maybe there are tasks that you don't want to do that you just can't avoid. But when you set out to have fun in the kitchen and create something you love, you're guaranteed pleasure and health. Three times a day, no matter where you live, you can make a conscious decision to exercise that right. By doing so, your body, mind, and spirit will thank you.

TIP

Still not inspired? Here are some tips to consider:

>> **Think about the advantages cooking at home could offer you.** Maybe it's saving money, eating healthier food, having a creative outlet, or something else.

>> **Think about what's missing from eating out in your area.** For example, many of my friends from overseas start cooking *more* when they come to the United States simply out of necessity, because they can't find foods from their homeland. Or maybe you have a dietary restriction that's hard for restaurants to accommodate.

>> **Pick an area (or two or three) around cooking that could be a fun challenge for you.** Maybe the idea of making the best use out of certain ingredients, repurposing leftovers, or making family recipes will inspire you.

REMEMBER

Effort in the kitchen is like everything else in life: The more you put in, the more you get out. If you relax and really allow yourself to *enjoy* the process — whether you're making toast or an elaborate masterpiece — you'll be grateful for the time you spend in the kitchen,

TIP

Cooking and using your hands is the perfect antidote for office and computer work. It allows you to get out of your head and into your senses and your dreams. The famous chef Julia Child once said, "Cooking is like love — it should be entered into with abandon or not at all." That's a very Mediterranean sentiment, and I promise that if you think of cooking that way, you'll have a lifelong companion that can keep you healthy and happy, just like love can.

Fitting cooking into your life

Just because people in the Mediterranean region value cooking, eating well, and communal meals, doesn't mean that they don't have anything else to do. With the exception of rural areas and the islands, most people have demanding jobs, families, and commutes to deal with nowadays. So being able to get fresh, wholesome meals on the table takes advance planning and effort.

TIP

You can use those some strategies to eat better wherever you live. It doesn't matter what your schedule is like or what kind of food you like to eat — there are a wide array of tricks that can make your time in the kitchen more efficient, including the following:

>> Figure out when you'll have a few hours at home in the next week and decide which of those hours would be best spent in the kitchen or when you'd be most inspired to cook.

>> Set up your pantry (see Chapter 14), your weekly menu (see Chapter 12), and your grocery list (see Chapter 15) ahead of time.

>> Decide when to go shopping, delegate the task, or have food delivered.

>> When you have your produce, wash it. Chop and prep vegetables (with the exception of onions) in advance — this way, you'll have everything ready when it's time to cook.

Different cooking styles work best for different lifestyles. Sometimes it varies from week to week. In that case, you can do a little planning each week based on what the week ahead will look like. The following sections cover some styles I find helpful.

The weekend warrior

This method of cooking and prep allows you to do the majority of the work in a two-hour block on the weekend (or whenever your most convenient day is) in order to have nutritious, homemade meals all week. With this approach, you're basically acting as your own personal chef. You decide in advance which vegetables and proteins you'd like to eat during the week and then make meals out of those ingredients in advance. At night, all you need to do is reheat them and serve with a fresh salad or side dish of your choice.

This option works extremely well for those who work very long days or have long commutes. When I first started my cooking and writing career, I had a very demanding job with a long commute, so this was a strategy that helped me immensely.

TIP

Here are some tips on making this approach work:

>> With a two-hour block of time, you can roast a chicken, roast a whole fish, roast a sheet pan with fish fillets and vegetables, and make an egg dish, such as a frittata. You can also use the stovetop to sauté vegetables and boil beans, legumes, grains, rice or pasta.

>> Make one meal out of the roasted whole fish and vegetables and salad for that night.

>> Place the other items — chicken, fish fillets, frittata, vegetables, legumes, and grains — in transparent containers and store in the refrigerator *or* make individual meal-size servings of each one for lunch and store in the refrigerator.

>> When you come home on busy evenings, simply combine a protein with a grain along with a vegetable and green salad, and you'll have a complete, delicious, and nutritious meal.

>> Eat the fish first, then the chicken, and then the egg, bean, and legume dishes, for the sake of freshness. If you don't plan on eating the chicken within three days, for example, you can freeze some of it so it'll stay fresher longer. Some people I know use the weekend warrior strategy once every two weeks, making a double portion of everything and freezing extras for the second week.

>> When your protein-based ingredients are used up, combine the remaining beans and legumes with vegetables and grains for the next night's dinners.

The improvisational cook

If you like the ritual of cooking a meal every night, but you're short on time, be sure to keep your ingredients prepped and ready to go for easy use. Keep containers of cooked grains, beans, lentils, and chopped produce ready to go in your refrigerator so when you come home at night you can toss them together in a way that you most enjoy while only waiting for the protein to cook.

FAST FOOD THE MEDITERRANEAN WAY

To me, fast food doesn't involve a drive-thru window, burgers, or fries. There's nothing wrong with those meals on occasion, but I need something I can rely on, something I enjoy, something that incudes genuine ingredients, connects me to my roots, and is good for me. This is when I turn to what I call "fast food my way," which is really the Mediterranean way.

Going on a road trip or traveling? Got a long commute? Most cooks work long hours and come home very late. I realized early in my teaching career that I couldn't afford (in terms of time or energy) to cook a "real" meal for myself at midnight when I got home from work. On occasion, I would turn to an improvisational Italian *spaghettata* (hot, al dente spaghetti tossed with good quality extra-virgin olive oil, garlic, chilies, and whatever else you like). But I didn't want to make that a daily habit, so I turned to other ingredients and recipes, like those in Chapter 18. I like to keep these items on hand specifically for these occasions.

Fast food could also be fresh, wholesome bread with cheese and grapes, a simple salad with a hard-boiled egg, whole-wheat pita with labneh or Greek yogurt drizzled with olive oil, and perhaps some cherry tomatoes or homemade hummus. I love salads of all stripes that can be quickly tossed together — I keep all the ingredients prepped in the fridge. Any variety of egg-based dishes are the kind of fast food that also save time, provide a nutrient and flavor boost, and are easy to make.

The hobbyist

This style of cooking is for people who enjoy cooking, but only when they can really lose themselves in the process and cook something truly special. For this type of cooking, I recommend creating very large portions when you cook — doubling or tripling a recipe. This way, you can portion it out and get more use out of it throughout the week, as well as freeze some for another time.

Feasting versus Fasting in the Mediterranean Region

Dietitians and nutritionists are often asked to create eating plans based around the Mediterranean diet for their clients. These eating plans are created with certain calorie restrictions and nutritional requirements to help people meet their health goals. This scientific approach, although effective, isn't always totally in line with the tenets of the Mediterranean lifestyle. Eating according to a set plan can also become monotonous.

Beginning in antiquity and continuing through today, diets in the Mediterranean region have never been static. People don't *always* eat the same types of foods and the same amounts day in and day out. Every culture has a religiously based fasting tradition. In turn, after the fasts, there is a period of feasting. The majority of the days are spent eating healthfully, but neither the Mediterranean lifestyle nor the Mediterranean diet require followers to eat a perfectly sugar- or carb-free diet year-round.

REMEMBER

Neither feasting nor fasting is a daily occurrence in the Mediterranean. Many Mediterranean diet enthusiasts are perplexed by the paradox of sugar-laden sweets such as baklava, the traditional sweet Italian breakfasts, and the ways that French fries seem to show up on tables everywhere. Eating a slice of baklava or a handful of fries in addition to a day's (or week's) worth of fresh, local foods prepared in healthful ways is not the worst thing in the world. Studies show that occasional indulgences like these are actually beneficial because they allow us to satisfy our desire for certain foods, making us feel fulfilled and content. The minute you deem foods as completely "off limits," you crave them — making it more difficult to stick to a solid eating plan.

In the following sections, I explain the concept of feasting and fasting, so you can incorporate *both* in your life.

Why feasts matter

Senza'a festa non si credi alli santi is a Calabrian phrase in dialect, which means "Without the feasts, no one believes in the saints." Feasting has followed fasting periods in the Mediterranean region since pagan times in antiquity. Many of those same traditions became part of the Christian, Jewish, and Muslim practices. Fast-forward thousands of years and people abstaining from foods for a certain amount of time and then preparing feasts has become a way of life.

Historically, feasts were times for communities to come together, to celebrate something in common, to socialize, and to share. Preparations for the festivities — whether they're religious or secular — give people a break from the mundane while providing a sense of security in the continuation of rituals that they've been doing their whole lives. Feasts create happiness and joy by dazzling the eyes with copious displays of carefully prepared foods and drinks. Psychologically, feasts help to remind us that bad times always end and that light and festivities are always found at the end of darkness and suffering.

The biggest feasts in the Mediterranean region occur on the most important religious holidays:

>> **Christianity:** Easter, Christmas, and various saints' days

>> **Islam:** Ramadan, the Eid al-Adha

>> **Judaism:** Rosh Hashanah and Yom Kippur

Other big feasts occur on equinox festivals, such as Egypt's The Smell of the Fresh Breeze festival and others. Feasts are also planned for welcoming important or out-of-town or country guests, for wedding ceremonies, and to celebrate other triumphs.

In terms of actual dishes, feasting foods in the region are always made up of the most coveted, seasonal items in large amounts. Labor-intensive breads, baked goods, and sweets that are too laborious and/or costly for daily consumption are also included. Often, the menus will include ingredients that people had to abstain from during their fasts. For example, on a Catholic holiday, mass is sure to be followed by a feast including meat. In the Greek Orthodox faith, which requires followers to follow a predominantly vegan diet during Lent, the Easter feast will include lots of dairy-rich foods and meats. Muslims who fast from sun up to sun down during Ramadan enjoy especially intricate and rich foods after they break their fast at sundown.

Fasting: An ancient ritual with modern appeal

Most modern medical texts and encyclopedias discuss fasting for medical reasons being prescribed by Hippocrates since the fifth century BCE. Fasting was being done in the spiritual world before that, however. To give thanks to what the Ancient Egyptians referred to as a Nile god named Hapi, they would place a roll of papyrus containing a prayer on the Nile. Osiri was the name of the agrarian god who was cast into the Nile and returned to life. The Ancient Egyptians drew a parallel between Hapi's resurrection and the growth of wheat that was sown into the ground previously flooded by the Nile. The Egyptians would also make offerings of fruits, vegetables, and flowers to show their appreciation for the Nile's rising. Prior to the festival, there was a period of fasting, in which people were forbidden from fishing, drinking water, or taking from the Nile. When celebrations began, however, dancing and singing would take place all night long, and people would drink water from the Nile. The joyous occasion of the Nile's rising in antiquity meant that fields of crops would be able to be irrigated year-round and that the citizens of Ancient Egypt would have enough to eat.

When American doctors set out to study the lifestyle habits of the healthiest Mediterranean populations in the mid-20th century, much of what they recorded was about people abstaining from meat and dairy. As a result, many Western doctors who prescribe the Mediterranean diet have become vegetarians and vegans themselves. But you don't need to become a vegetarian or vegan in order to follow the lifestyle and diet accurately.

TECHNICAL STUFF

The reason why so many people appeared not to eat meat when they were being studied was due to religious fasts. The Greek Orthodox community fasts 180 to 200 days per year. During this time, they follow a vegetarian or vegan diet. What you can take away from this practice is not the importance of giving up meat completely, but how not eating it all the time and living mostly off of plant-based foods, just like the Mediterranean Diet Pyramid recommends, is a great idea. (Turn to Chapter 13 for more on the pyramid.)

In the Roman Catholic traditions, fasts are still widely observed, especially at a culinary level, when meat is abstained from on Fridays and is traditionally not eaten until Sunday after having the Eucharist at mass. Fasting also occurred at different times during the year and on saints' days, although those are no longer as common, especially with the general population. In addition to the meatless Fridays of Lent, there is a popular custom of "giving up something" that the believer truly enjoys. This way, you feel a bit of suffering similar to the suffering of Jesus.

The Jewish faith has six observed fasting days in which food is abstained from morning to night. A full Jewish fast lasts from sunset to sundown the following night. There are two Jewish full fast days — Tisha B'Av and Yom Kippur (the only fast day mentioned in the Torah) — as well as minor fasting days of Fast of Gedalia (Tzom Gedalia), Tenth of Tevet (Asara B'Tevet), Seventeenth of Tammuz (Shiva Asar B'Tammuz), and the Fast of Esther (Ta'anit Esther). The two full fast days include additional restrictions in addition to eating and drinking. For example, you aren't allowed to wash your body; wear leather shoes; use colognes, oils, or perfumes; or have sex. Yom Kippur also has the same restrictions of Shabbat (the Sabbath), and Tisha B'Av has different restrictions somewhat similar to a mourner in the Jewish tradition.

Ramadan is the month on the Islamic lunar calendar when Muslims fast from sun up to sundown each day in order to attain self-discipline and piety. Muslims believe that Ramadan is the month when the Torah, the New Testament, and the Koran were revealed to mankind. Although Ramadan is a difficult time of physical fasting, it's also a very beloved month by those who observe it because it's the time of the kitchen and family. In the evenings, after the fast is broken, people get together, socializing and praying. In addition to abstaining from food, no negative talk, slandering, swearing, or "impure" acts are permitted during Ramadan. Muslims believe that Allah recognizes and counts the good deeds of a Muslim more during the month of Ramadan and that their sins are also multiplied. The fast is not considered complete until an obligatory charity is paid at the end. Many Muslims also fast one or two days a week and on other holy days in order to remain spiritually fit.

REMEMBER

Abstaining from eating is only *one* component of fasting. Spiritual fasts help people to retrain their minds and foster positive, healthful thoughts. Long before therapy and psychoanalysis were a part of our lives, people in the Mediterranean were using fasting to achieve the best versions of themselves.

For people who have grown up with fasting as a part of their culture, it's a rewarding and appreciated experience. For those who have not, it can be quite daunting in the beginning! I remember when I first made the decision that I wanted to fast during the month of Ramadan. I had so much difficulty in the beginning, until I mentioned it to a Jewish friend. She said, "Amy, abstaining from food is about mind over matter. We also fast in our faith, and I have to mentally prepare myself before doing so. I remind myself why this is a healthful practice for me, and why I want to do it. Once you can do that, you will have no problem." She was right. I took her advice, and from then on, I was able to use spiritual fasts as a means of achieving peace.

I've found that when I abstain from food and drink for an entire day, my mind becomes much freer. It's difficult to "sweat the small stuff" when you're hungry. A month long of fasting for me, even though I was working full time, provided much-needed mental breaks from stress and unnecessary suffering.

Ancient Traditions for Modern-Day Results

Intermittent fasting is a buzz term that continues to get more and more press. I first learned about it from my dear friend and culinary medicine partner Dr. Sam Pappas, who prescribes various types of fasts to his patients to help them achieve their health goals. Although many modern fasts have nothing to do with spirituality per se, Dr. Pappas draws upon his Greek roots to find deeper meaning and significance with them for his patients. The various styles of fasting have been proven to help lose and maintain weight, improve digestion, and improve or reverse certain health conditions and help us adapt to hormonal and life changes.

WARNING

Be sure to consult a doctor before embarking upon intermittent fasting in order to achieve the best results.

Popular methods of intermittent fasting include the following:

>> **The 16/8 method:** You skip breakfast and restrict your daily eating period to 8 hours, such as noon to 8 p.m. Then you fast for 16 hours in between.

>> **The 5:2 diet:** You consume only 500 to 600 calories on two nonconsecutive days of the week, but you eat normally the other five days.

>> **Eat-stop-eat:** You fast for 24 hours, once or twice a week (for example, by not eating from dinner one day until dinner the next day).

>> **Alternate-day fasting:** You fast every other day. Some interpretations allow about 500 calories on the fasting days; others do not.

>> **Warrior diet:** You eat small amounts of raw fruits and vegetables during the day and eat one huge meal at night, usually within a four-hour eating window.

>> **Spontaneous meal skipping:** You skip a meal here or there when you aren't hungry or you're traveling. This approach works for people who don't need to eat three meals a day in order to maintain muscle mass and even blood sugar levels.

REMEMBER

Intermittent fasting isn't for everyone. If you want to try it, talk with your doctor before you start. Eating fewer meals means you really need to pay attention to the nutrients you're getting when you do eat, so be sure to pack in as much flavor and good-for-you ingredients as you can when you eat.

If you're fasting on a regular basis, you've got fewer opportunities to nourish yourself with the vitamins, minerals, and pleasure of eating than you normally would. For that reason, it's extremely important to keep both pleasure and health at the forefront. Make sure that what you *do* eat is something you love and that it provides the same amount of affection back to your heart, mind, body, and spirit.

The art of DIY

The pride that people take in making things with their own hands in the Mediterranean region is a critical part of the Mediterranean lifestyle. Obviously, no one has an unlimited amount of time, and modern cultures are set up to enable people to be able to buy whatever they like and need. That said, many people like to make things with their own hands — from arts and crafts, to pottery, to woodworking or furniture, to knitting . . . it really doesn't matter. The point is that creating things on your own gives you a sense of completion and accomplishment, as well as being a pleasurable pastime that helps to release hormones and neurotransmitters that help you feel better.

In the Mediterranean region, the number-one way of celebrating the DIY attitude is with food. If you're invited to someone's home for dinner, whether it's in Egypt, Greece, Italy, or somewhere else, your host will most likely share the origin of the food and their connection to it. You may hear, "I grew these vegetables in my garden," "This extra-virgin olive oil is from my uncle's orchard," "This is one of the chickens that we raise," "Those apples are from the tree in our backyard," or "We pickle these vegetables, dry those peppers, and cure that meat ourselves." The list of comments like that from just a week's worth of eating with friends and family could fill this entire chapter!

Doing things yourself is important because, in addition to the pleasure it provides, it ensures better quality control. If you're cooking with food that is local and making it yourself, it'll be better for you because you'll put better-quality ingredients into it than large companies who are manufacturing things in the most cost-effective and shelf-stable way possible.

If you're raising your own vegetables or animals, you know how you're caring for them, what they're eating, and when they were harvested or slaughtered. Pickling your own fruits and vegetables — even from a nearby farm or farmers market is better than buying them from a store if you have the opportunity. Obviously, most people can't just stop their lives to make sure they're doing everything themselves. What you can do, however, is pick the items that mean the most to you and start there.

When I was living in a place where I couldn't have a garden and didn't have much space, I had to be really picky about what I grew, so I chose herbs and Calabrian chili peppers. I could harvest them in pots, and I used to string the herbs and peppers separately and hang them on my bedroom window sill to dry. I would then put the herbs into jars for my nightly tisanes, and the peppers, once dry, I ground in a coffee grinder that I used just for that purpose and stored in jars. Neither of those DIY projects took up a significant amount of time or space, but by doing them I was able to use ingredients that are important to me and my heritage on a daily basis, which I grew and harvested myself. I saved money and got better results, and so can you!

TIP

You can start with one teeny project, like herbs, and find a passion that will improve your health and cooking. Here are some tips if you want to try your hand at some DIY kitchen projects:

>> Decide which ingredients you use daily and couldn't live without, and pick one or two to focus on. Say your favorite staple food is coffee — you can start out by grinding and brewing your own coffee every day.

>> If you love pottery, enroll in a class to learn how to make your own or even paint your own. Be sure to create some pieces that you'll use on a daily basis.

>> Start an herb or vegetable garden. All you need is a windowsill!

>> Plant some fruit trees. If you don't have a yard, go to a farm to pick produce. It's fun and the quality is better. Then make something with your harvest.

>> Commit to replacing one of your favorite jarred items — a sauce, a dressing, an herb or spice mix — and begin making it on your own. You can make it in large batches and store it for daily use.

THE ROLE OF AGRICULTURE

Agricultural crops grew abundantly in the Nile Valley during ancient times, thanks to the rising of the Nile. Beans, cucumbers, dates, figs, garlic, grapes, juniper, leeks, lemons, lentils, mint, peas, plums, and pomegranates all flourished. The Ancient Egyptians ate a wide variety of meats, poultry, and fish. They used food to nourish their minds, bodies, and spirits.

If we want to be truly healthy — not only individually but as a society — we need to make a commitment to support sustainable farming and secure the solid future of agriculture. By embracing the strategies used by our great-grandparents, we'll be able to avoid the epidemic of modern food scarcity.

Here are some ways we can use successful sustainable agricultural practices to improve our health:

* We can support legislation that promotes good, clean, fair farming.

* We can join organizations such as Slow Food (www.slowfood.com) that promote good, clean, fair food at a global level.

* We can determine with our doctors which nutritional supplements would be best for us, given our blood tests, diets, and medicine usage.

* We can join community-supported agriculture (CSA) organizations, shop at farmers markets, and support farmers as often as possible.

4 Preparing and Eating Food with Pleasure

Chapter **12**

Ancient Flavor Enhancers and Plant-Based Menus

This chapter is about bringing more flavor to your meals through aromatics, like onions, garlic, herbs, and spices. I also fill you in on how to come up with plant-based menus and how to cook with the seasons.

Adding Flavor with Aromatics

If you're interested in adding flavor to your dishes without adding more salt or fat, meet your new best friend: aromatics. *Aromatics* are key ingredients that enhance the flavor of dishes. They include vegetables, fruits, alliums (such as onions, garlic, leeks, and chives), as well as fresh herbs and spices. You can combine these ingredients in a multitude of ways and use a variety of cooking styles. In addition, each of these ingredients offers nutritional benefits, which act as culinary medicine for the body. Every time you add them to your dishes, you can be assured that you're increasing the flavor; decreasing fat, calories, and sodium; and gaining the benefits of powerful nutrients.

When you know how to work with aromatics, you have the keys to great flavor and optimal health. Spices and herbs have been used for centuries for their great taste and nutritional benefits. From sweet and floral to hot and spicy, just changing the type of pepper you use can change your entire meal.

Why flavor matters

Mediterranean culinary cultures place just as much emphasis on flavor as they do on health. When you eat flavorful foods, you're more satisfied — both physically and emotionally. Foods that are full of flavor fill you up more quickly and prevent you from making unhealthful food choices. Many of them have powerful antioxidant and anti-inflammatory properties as well, which makes them a natural choice upon which to build the foundations of flavor.

Many of the flavor enhancers that we use nowadays — such as garlic, onions, herbs, and spices — have been around since ancient times. Others, like peppers, are recent additions from the Americas. Regardless of their source, however, they've all been adapted to the local cuisines to the point that it's difficult to imagine our favorite dishes without them.

Here are some of the most popular aromatics in the Mediterranean region:

>> **Bell peppers:** Green, red, orange, and purple bell peppers are used throughout the Mediterranean region. As flavor enhancers, they're often sautéed in olive oil alongside onions and garlic, or with the ubiquitous trinity of onions, celery, and carrots.

>> **Carrots:** Carrots are used in conjunction with celery and onions at the initial stage of cooking in recipes. In addition to the health benefits that they offer, they add sweetness, crunch or creaminess, and color to recipes.

>> **Celery:** Celery has a high moisture content and is believed to lower blood pressure when consumed in large quantities. Although it was grown in the Mediterranean for millennia, it was a latecomer to the United States. In fact, a century ago, celery was so hard to come by in the United States that it was considered a delicacy and served on its own in special dishes at White House dinners. Nowadays, we take celery for granted, but in the Mediterranean it's used extensively as part of a flavor-building mixture in the beginning of recipes. Even celery leaves can add great flavor and nutritional benefits to cooking.

>> **Chili peppers:** Although not indigenous to the Mediterranean region, chili peppers are so popular that billboards welcoming you to the Southern Italian region of Calabria prominently display them. They can be dried and crushed, eaten fresh, made into pastes, or sautéed as a flavor foundation. Various types of chili peppers can add heat, smokiness, and depth of flavor to your dishes.

>> **Garlic:** Garlic is nature's antibiotic. Many people in the Mediterranean region eat raw cloves of garlic to prevent illness. In the kitchen, garlic is used raw in pesto, hummus, baba ghanouj, and many other dishes. It's also sautéed to varying degrees of doneness, usually in extra-virgin olive oil, and served as a condiment to everything from pasta to vegetables to fish and meat.

>> **Herbs:** Herbs have been used both in cooking and for healing purposes since antiquity in the Mediterranean region. In modern cities such as Rome, Athens, and Tel Aviv, you can find herbalists who sell various wellness-boosting herbs. Flavor profiles range from country to country, but fresh parsley, basil, cilantro, dill, mint, marjoram, rosemary, sage, and thyme are all used in copious amounts. Many of the herbs are also dried to make hot infusions known as *tisanes,* which are enjoyed before bed or when someone is sick or dieting.

>> **Leeks:** Roman soldiers were fed leeks in order to stay strong and healthy, and we can use them today for the same reason. In cooking, leeks add a deeper flavor that helps to round out and brighten soups and stews.

>> **Onions:** Onions are the unsung heroes of the kitchen. Depending on the variety and how they're cooked, they can add sweetness, sharpness, creaminess, or crunch to a recipe. From slowly simmered onions that create the creamy backbone to risotto dishes in Italy, to the dark-golden, deep-fried onions that top Egyptian lentils and rice, onions are integral to flavor. Various sizes and colors have varying health benefits, but in general, onions help rid the body's cells of waste material.

>> **Shallots:** Shallots are milder in flavor than onions. They're believed to promote weight maintenance and help prevent blood sugar levels from spiking, and they're used extensively in Southern France and the Levant. You can pan-fry shallots in extra-virgin olive oil and use them as a garnish for vegetables, soups, rice dishes, and stews. They can also be roasted whole, alongside vegetables or protein, or quartered and braised in stock.

>> **Spices:** Spices are used sparingly in the Southern European portion of the Mediterranean and more extensively in the Levant and North African regions. Chapter 14 explains how to use cinnamon, ginger, turmeric, cumin, chili, black pepper, cloves, nutmeg, coriander, saffron, sumac, smoked paprika, and sea salts for maximum flavor and health benefits.

>> **Vanilla:** Vanilla is an important flavor enhancer because it can trick the taste buds into thinking that you're eating something sweet. Add a little extra vanilla to a chocolate recipe, and the chocolate flavor will intensify. Using a bit more vanilla in baking enables you to cut down on the sugar because the brain associates vanilla with sweetness.

How to use aromatics in your dishes

In the Mediterranean, many of a cook's "secret techniques" lie within their use of aromatics. For thousands of years, housewives and professional chefs alike had nothing to flavor their food with other than aromatics. Nowadays, sugar, salt, and fat are cheap and readily available. For this reason, restaurant chefs and home cooks turn to them repeatedly to add flavor to food. But in the Mediterranean, that wasn't always the case. Consider the following:

>> **Sugar:** Up until about a hundred years ago, sugar was too expensive to use on a regular basis. The French, for example, used to go to apothecaries to get a tablespoon at a time when they were sick, in order to relieve their maladies. Therefore, sweets couldn't be eaten on a daily basis and were reserved for special occasions. Plus, people couldn't just add a little sweetness to their food by increasing the sugar content. They had to find other ways to enhance the sweetness of their sauces and desserts.

>> **Salt:** Throughout history, salt was either very expensive on its own or highly taxed, For that reason, there were no salt shakers at tables and cooks didn't have the luxury of adding as much salt as they wanted. So — you guessed it — they had to come up with other solutions to enhance their culinary creations.

>> **Fat:** People have always used fat to flavor foods, but the types of fat that we use today are different from those that were used historically. In the Mediterranean region, head-to-tail butchering was a necessity, not a trend. If an animal was slaughtered, every portion of it was used, and fat would be rendered from the less desirable parts of the animal to make a sort of rudimentary lard. This type of fat, along with extra-virgin olive oil were the main sources of fat-based flavoring in the Mediterranean region throughout history, and they are today as well.

Fast-forward to our modern kitchens. You can stock your cupboards with lentils, beans, barley, and other grains, as well as herbs and spices. Your refrigerator can be full of fresh vegetables.

TIP

Now, how do you go about cooking those ingredients in a manner that allows you to coax the most flavor from them? Here are my tips:

>> **Build a flavor base.** Whether they're referred to by a specific name (such as the Spanish *sofrito,* French *mirepoix,* Italian *soffrito*) or not, all Mediterranean countries use aromatics in various proportions to layer flavors in their food.

>> **Use aromatics as swap-outs.** Want to add more of a salty flavor to your dishes without increasing the sodium content? Try tossing in some fresh baby dill (it's full of mineral salts) or, for slowly simmered dishes, try adding dried porcini mushrooms to add a depth of minerally flavor, which mimics salt. For added flavor without the fat or calories, onions, garlic, shallots, herbs, and spices are your best choices.

>> **Build better garnishes.** I'm a firm believer that garnishes play a strong role in a dish's overall flavor. Why settle for a sprig of parsley or a simple basil leaf when you can combine finely chopped herbs in larger quantities, add a drizzle of good-quality extra-virgin olive oil, or add a generous portion of caramelized onions, for example? The right garnish can take a recipe to new heights and add a lot of nutritional benefits.

>> **Create mouthwatering and nutritious stocks.** In my cooking classes, one of the first things I teach students is how to make stock. It may sound boring, but you can improve your cooking and health greatly by simply switching from commercial stocks to homemade ones. Traditional Mediterranean cooks always have them on hand to whip up a quick soup or risotto or add flavor to sauces, vegetables, and rice dishes.

>> **Transform pantry items into meals.** Many people have rice, pasta, beans, legumes, and spices in their pantries. Although this book suggests having a slightly larger pantry, even those four simple ingredients with the help of aromatics can be transformed into a simple, satisfying, and nutritious meal in less time than it takes to order delivery. Most Mediterranean countries have their own versions of lentils and/or beans and rice and pasta and lentils and/or beans. One-dish dinners including skillets, soups, pastas, and salads can be prepared with the help of aromatics.

TIP

Keep these decadent and nutritionally potent recipes on hand:

>> ***Ras el hanout* spice mixture:** *Ras el hanout* means "head of the shop" in Arabic. A version I tasted at a spice shop in Tangiers had 57 different spice mixes in it. Spice mixes are an integral part of Moroccan cuisine, and many people claim that their version is best. This is a great mixture to add to soups, stews, tajines, roasted vegetables, and anything you want to give depth of flavor to without adding fat or calories. The cumin, ginger, and cinnamon all have wonderful anti-inflammatory properties.

In a bowl, combine the following ingredients, and stir until combined:

- 2 teaspoons ground cumin

- 2 teaspoons ground ginger

- 3 teaspoons kosher salt or sea salt

- 2 teaspoons freshly ground black pepper

- 2 teaspoons ground cinnamon

- 1 teaspoon ground coriander

- ¼ teaspoon ground cloves

- ¼ teaspoon ground cardamom

- ¼ teaspoon cayenne

- 1 teaspoon all-spice

- 1 teaspoon saffron

Place in an airtight container inside a cupboard and away from heat for up to 1 month.

» **Spanish *bravas*-style seasoning:** Keep this delicious mixture on hand for making paella or sprinkling on fried potatoes, seafood, and vegetables. Store this spice mix, along with other red spices, in airtight containers in the refrigerator for maximum flavor.

In a small, airtight container, combine the following ingredients:

- ¼ cup sweet paprika

- 1 teaspoon saffron

- ¼ teaspoon crushed red chili pepper

- 1 tablespoon unrefined sea salt

Store in the refrigerator for up to 1 year.

» **Za'taar (wild thyme spice mix):** *Za'taar* is the name of both wild thyme and a spice mix made with wild thyme in the Middle East. Particularly popular in Lebanon, za'taar is great for sprinkling on pita chips, yogurt, cheese, breads, and plain pizza dough. Some people like to dip fresh, hot pita bread in olive oil and then in za'taar. The combination of olive oil and this spice mix is given to people with respiratory illnesses.

In an airtight container, combine the following ingredients:

- ¼ cup dried ground za'taar (wild thyme) or regular dried thyme

- ¼ cup dried ground coriander

- ¼ cup sesame seeds

- 1 tablespoon dried ground cumin

- 1 tablespoon anise seeds
- 1 tablespoon fennel seeds
- 1 tablespoon sea salt

Shake well to combine, seal, and store in a dark, cool place for up to a year.

Finding Plant-Based Menus

According to the traditional Mediterranean style of eating, there is nothing wrong with the consumption of meat, and many people in the region would eat meat when they could. When it wasn't a time of religious fasting, when a special occasion was being celebrated, when a guest was being honored, or when it was the season to slaughter an animal, meat would be consumed. In the last century, the price of meat made it "off-limits" for families in various Mediterranean countries at different times, not because they didn't want to eat it, but because they couldn't afford it. As resources and wealth increased in the late 20th century and the region became more influenced by the West, more meat and poultry were added into daily diets. Many modern Mediterranean homes now serve more meat and poultry than they did before, because it's more affordable and readily available in most places.

Before the 1950s, people didn't plan their menus around their source of protein. They planned their daily meals based upon what was ripe in their gardens. (Many people in the Mediterranean still eat this way.) They made the most out of whatever they had. Although in many places people didn't realize the importance of this aspect for their own health, it was one of the best predicaments that Mother Nature could have put them in.

You can find all kinds of tips on how to incorporate more fruits and vegetables into your snacks or "sneak" them into your diet, but I prefer the option of just starting out by planning menus centered around fruits and vegetables. This way, you'll be sure to get enough of the good stuff every day, and snacks can be a way to get even more nutrients instead of making up for what your meals are missing.

Many Americans grew up with a "meat and potatoes" mentality. There's nothing wrong with meat and potatoes once in a while. But the traditional Mediterranean diet promotes eating smaller amounts of meat less frequently than a standard American diet does.

The second hurdle for many Americans to overcome when they're creating plant-focused menus is that they don't find a lot of inspiration in restaurants. Most modern restaurants feature the same "protein and carb" formula that was popular decades ago. Even if they offer vegetarian dishes, they tend to focus more on pantry staples (such as pasta) and less on fresh vegetables. For this reason, just thinking about transforming vegetables into lunch or dinner (with the exception of large salads) intimidates many American chefs and home cooks.

Because many people now rely on restaurants and freezer sections for the majority of their meals, it's really important to think about the best ways to incorporate some of the ancient wisdom for ourselves and our families. By making traditional menus, you can stay on top of your nutritional goals while enjoying yourself in the process.

Making traditional Mediterranean menus

In a typical Mediterranean meal, you can easily consume three to four servings of plant-based foods. Most traditional menus from the region contain even more than that. For millennia, meals were based around what produce was seasonal and available. Meat and dairy-based products were added to supplement the fruits and vegetables, not the other way around. By adopting this ancient approach to modern menus, you can make sure you're getting more nutrients than you would by eating meat-based menus with just a bit of produce.

One of the best parts about making traditional Mediterranean menus is that there are so many different styles to choose from! People in the different countries around the Mediterranean basin eat different styles of meals. Americans tend to think of a meal in terms of one plate (where you have a main course and one or two sides, all on one plate), but people in Southern Europe think in terms of courses, while those in North Africa and the Levant region tend to serve several dishes at once.

Generally speaking, most people eat their largest caloric intake in the middle of the day, not in the evening, so lunches (even if they're much later than those in the United States) are more abundant. Dinners usually come much later than dinners do in the United States — usually at 8 p.m. or later — and tend to be simple, unless it's a special occasion. Breakfast is what varies the most across the region; people in the South of France, Spain, and Italy usually opt for lighter breakfasts consisting of bread or morning pastries and juice, whereas North African and Levantine breakfasts include eggs, beans, pastrami, salad, fresh fruit, and more. In Egypt, Lebanon, and Israel for example, even falafel and tahini sauce are part of the breakfast menu.

There is an Italian proverb that translates as "Breakfast like a king, lunch like a prince, and dinner like a poor person," and if I had to sum up Mediterranean dining patterns in one phrase, I think that fits.

Putting produce front and center

Close your eyes and think back to some of your favorite dishes that contain fruits and vegetables. Hearty soups and stews, savory salads, savory pies and quiches, risotto, pilafs, pasta dishes, frittatas, and omelets usually come to mind. With a few "base recipes" up your sleeve, you can cook from the hip with vegetables easily and enjoyably.

TIP

In addition to side dishes, salads, and crudités with dips for an appetizer or snack, which are always great, here are some of my favorite ways to convert vegetable dishes into tantalizing main events:

>> **Soups:** Hearty, creamy purees and broth-based soups

>> **Egg dishes:** Frittatas, omelets, tortillas, and *shakshouka* (a popular egg, tomato, and pepper-based dish)

>> **Pasta dishes:** Everything from quick skillet dishes to layered lasagne

>> **One-dish wonders:** Gratins, casseroles, savory pies, and stews

>> **Fast, casual bowls, burritos, tacos, and wraps**

>> **Pizza, calzones, empanadas, *pides* (Turkish-style flatbreads), pitas, and *boreks* (savory filled dough pastries)**

>> **Smoothies and juice cocktails**

>> **Sweet breads and desserts:** Zucchini bread, banana bread, fruit bread, fruit-based pies and desserts, and puddings

Many of the recipes in this book can be varied to accommodate fridge foraging and repurposing leftovers. Challenge yourself to come up with the most intriguing leftover-based meals. After a few tries you won't even need a recipe, and you'll be on your way to thinking and cooking like someone in the Mediterranean.

TIP

Spend 30 minutes a week preparing your vegetables. With the exception of onions, everything can be washed, dried, cut, or sliced in advance. Then store those items in clear plastic containers with lids and stack them in the refrigerator.

If you have diced celery, diced carrots, chopped tomatoes, fresh corn kernels, clean baby spinach, chopped lettuce, clean and cut broccoli and cauliflower flowerets, all prepped and stored, even if you come home from a busy day at work or need to get a meal on the table fast, you can quickly put a meal together with a few of the pantry items from Chapter 14.

One night, for example, you could combine all the vegetables to create a large salad — perhaps topped with a hardboiled egg or leftover protein or a handful of crushed almonds or walnuts. Another meal could be made out of sautéing the carrots and celery with a freshly diced onion and olive oil; then add the rest of the produce and cover with water or stock. Bring to a boil, reduce the heat to low, and simmer until the vegetables are tender. Season with salt and pepper, and stir in a handful of your favorite herbs. For a creamy soup, that mixture could be pureed; for a regular soup, you could add a little more liquid to make it thinner. You could also add in pasta, rice or another grain, and beans or legumes to make a heartier soup.

Another option is to sauté some onion and garlic in extra-virgin olive oil in a large skillet; add the mixture of vegetables that you like best; season with salt, pepper, and a handful of fresh herbs; cover; and cook on low until the vegetables are tender. You can toss them with pasta or rice, or use them as a filling for frittatas, omelets, and more. You could also make some indentations with a spoon in the vegetable mixture and crack eggs into them. The combination of eggs and the right vegetables will provide you with the nutrients of a complete meal.

TIP

If you're a fan of the fast-casual restaurant concept, you can do the same thing with your refrigerator. In addition to the vegetables, prepare a few servings of whole grains in advance; rice, quinoa, pasta, barley, and wild rice are great choices. Keep a few cups of cooked lentils and cooked beans on hand in the refrigerator as well, along with chopped hardboiled eggs and/or a grilled or leftover protein of your choice. When you need a meal fast, you can make a bowl out of the combination of carbohydrate, protein, vegetables, and beans or legumes. Drizzle with extra-virgin olive oil and fresh citrus juice or vinegar. The same ingredients could be used in *lavash bread* (a Middle Eastern flatbread) or another thin bread to make a Mediterranean-style wrap, or in taco shells or tortillas. (Sure, those last two options aren't Mediterranean in origin, but they'll add variety to your diet and enable you to get more mileage out of your already prepped vegetables.)

Cooking with the Seasons

Our bodies were designed to need and crave the nutrients found in the produce that grows locally in the areas where we live. For example, if you live on the East Coast of the United States, your body will benefit much more from eating fresh, local berries in June than it will from eating a frozen version in December. Technically speaking, a strawberry's nutritional value doesn't vary from place to place.

The soil, however, does vary, and our bodies need the nutrients that fruits and vegetables get from the soil where we live.

That said, growing vegetables in your own garden, shopping in farmers markets, participating in a community-supported agriculture (CSA) program, or choosing fresh and local produce from your supermarket has many advantages to it. These items are cheaper than those that come from far away. Plus, they reduce your carbon footprint and are excellent for your health.

TIP

Eating seasonally helps you to enjoy a wide variety of vitamins and minerals and stretches your culinary creativity (see the nearby sidebar).

REMEMBER

What grows together goes together. This saying can refer to a wine and olive oil pairing or to produce. In the springtime where I live, for example, fennel, dandelion greens, spring herbs, and spring vegetables are all in season, and they taste fresh, bright, and satisfying when paired together. Likewise, the tomatoes, eggplant, and zucchini of late summer are perfect partners, as are the squash, mushrooms, and woody herbs of the fall season.

GETTING CREATIVE IN THE KITCHEN

In the Mediterranean region, any chef or home cook worth their salt knows at least dozens of recipes to make with every vegetable that grows in their area. A Turkish chef once told me that he wouldn't hire anyone for his team unless they could cook eggplant at least 40 different ways. Years ago, young brides supposedly needed to know how to do the same. The reason for this is that when people had gardens, they lived off of what they grew. People gave thanks for their sustenance and didn't have the option to buy other ingredients, so they made the best out of what they had.

Nowadays, even the most remote places in the Mediterranean region have supermarkets. Locals, however, view them as a means to supplement what they grow, not as a substitute for a garden. When I spend time in Ikaria, Greece, I'm always impressed to see everyone gardening. Instead of going to the grocery store, most residents barter with their neighbors to increase their variety of ingredients. This is a wonderful and healthy goal for our world as well.

If you're not acquainted with what's in season where you live, here are some suggestions:

>> **Enroll in a CSA program.** The fruits and vegetables that you get in your CSA box will be grown locally, which means, by definition, they're what's in season where you live.

>> **Shop at farmers markets.** Here you not only get the fruits and vegetables that are in season, but you get a chance to talk with the farmers (or their staff) about their produce. They may be able to offer suggestions on how to cook their foods, too.

>> **Grow as many of your own produce as you can.** If you can grow it in your yard, it's in season! Don't have a yard? You can grow many things in containers on a balcony or patio.

Chapter **13**

Planning Meals with the Mediterranean Diet Pyramid

This chapter introduces the Mediterranean Diet Pyramid, a visual guide to the Mediterranean lifestyle. It explains which types of foods should be eaten when and helps you plan menus using the pyramid as a guide. Unlike many Mediterranean meal planners on the market, it doesn't give typical American meal items with swapped-out Mediterranean ingredients. Instead, in this chapter, you see what people eat in the Mediterranean and why, so you can participate in lifestyle rituals that have stood the test of time.

Understanding the Mediterranean Diet Pyramid

In 1993, the nonprofit organization Oldways created the Mediterranean Diet Pyramid (see Figure 13-1) in partnership with the Harvard School of Public Health and the World Health Organization as a healthier alternative to the USDA's original food pyramid.

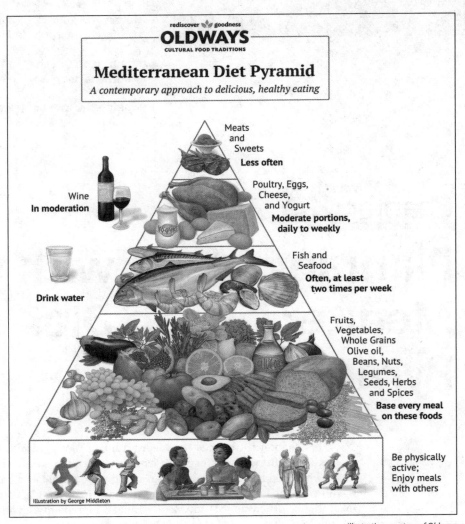

FIGURE 13-1:
The Mediterranean
Diet Pyramid.

Illustration courtesy of Oldways

**TECHNICAL
STUFF**

The Mediterranean Diet Pyramid is a modern invention to help people make healthful Mediterranean choices on their own. In the Mediterranean region, of course, the local cultures promote this style of eating without any pyramids — it's just the way they live.

REMEMBER

In order to fully benefit from the Mediterranean lifestyle, you need to focus on more than just diet alone. By taking a positive attitude toward food (instead of looking at it as a problem to be solved), you'll be able to appreciate the important role it plays in the Mediterranean lifestyle. Throughout the region, food is viewed not only as a traditional medicinal, but also as a form of artistic expression, a

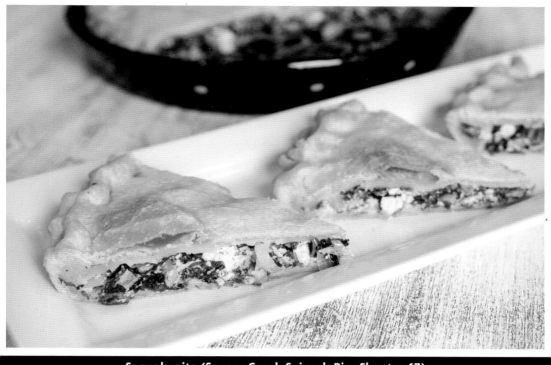

Spanakopita (Savory Greek Spinach Pie; Chapter 17)

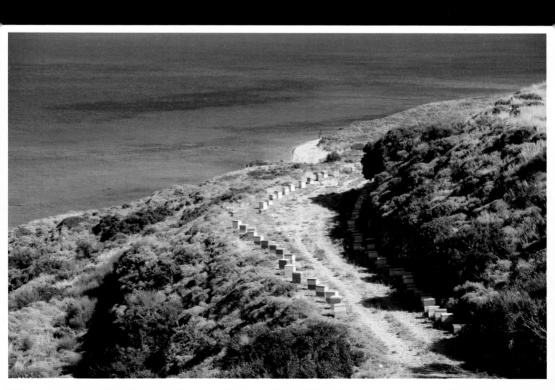

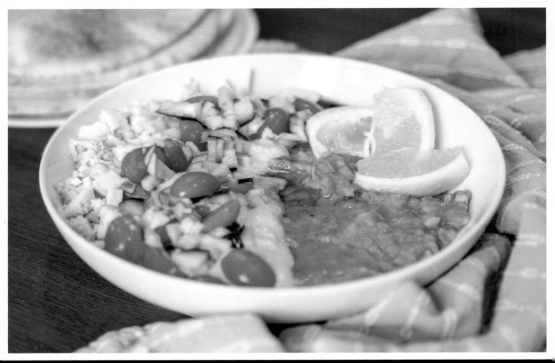

Egyptian Fuul Medammes with Tahini (Chapter 17)

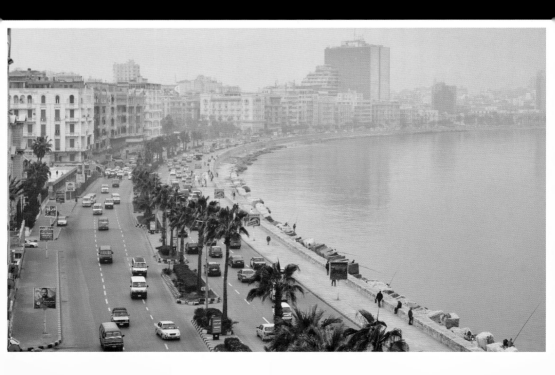

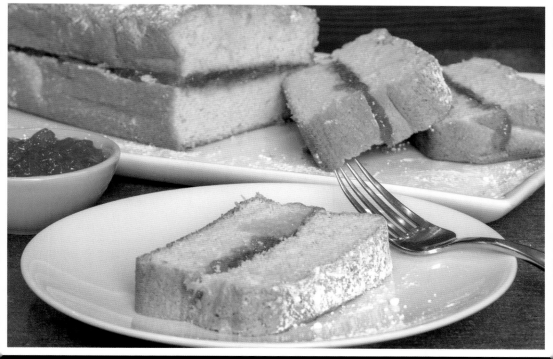

Pan di Spagna (Italian Sponge Cake; Chapter 17)

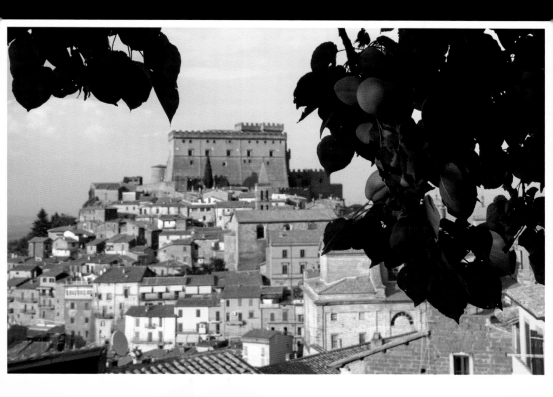

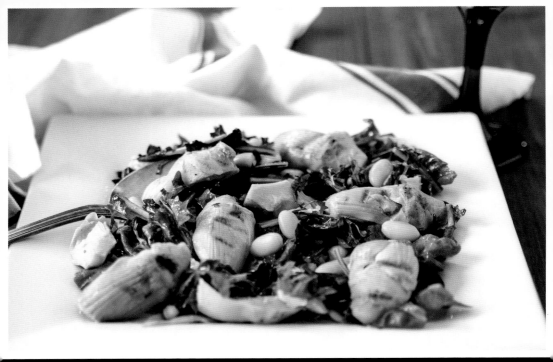

Cannellini Beans with Artichoke Hearts and Dandelion Greens (Chapter 18)

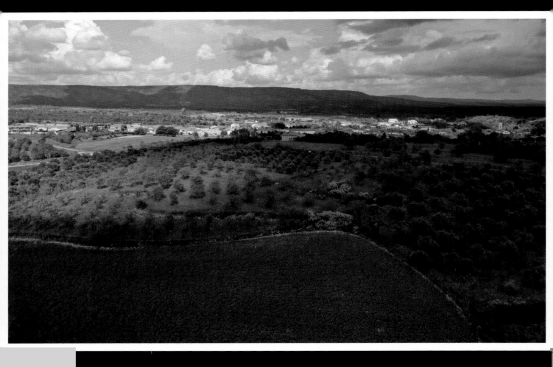

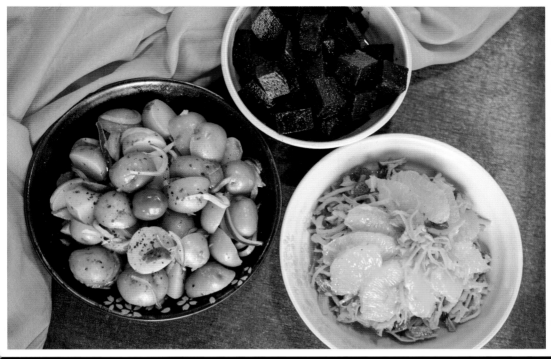

Moroccan Vegetable Salad Sampler (Chapter 18)

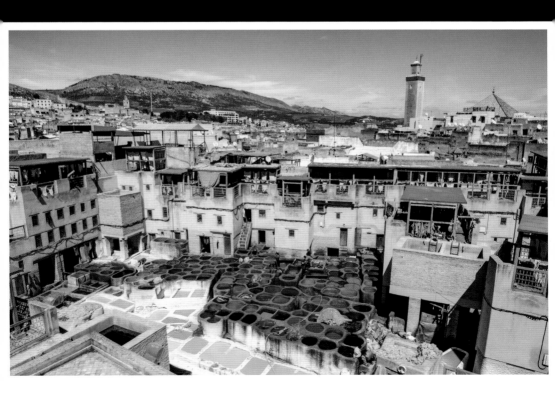

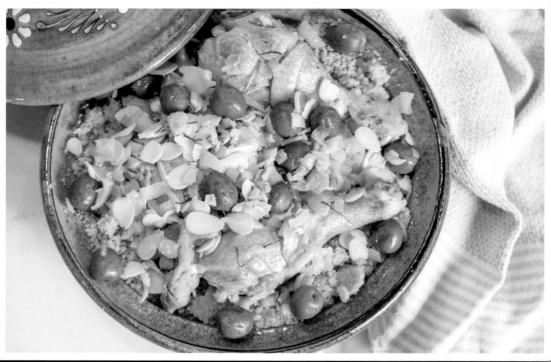

Tajine Djaj bil Couscous (Moroccan Chicken, Almond, and Olive Tajine with Couscous; Chapter 19)

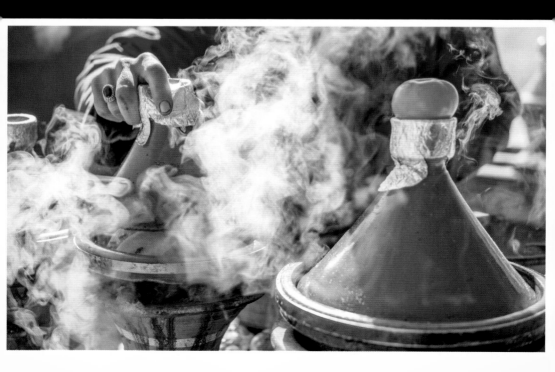

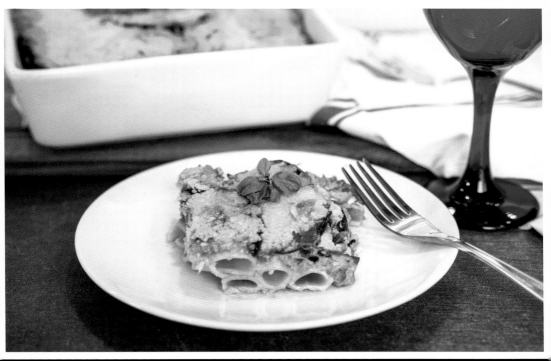

Pasta al Forno con Melanzane e Caciocavallo (Baked Pasta with Eggplant and Caciocavallo; Chapter 19)

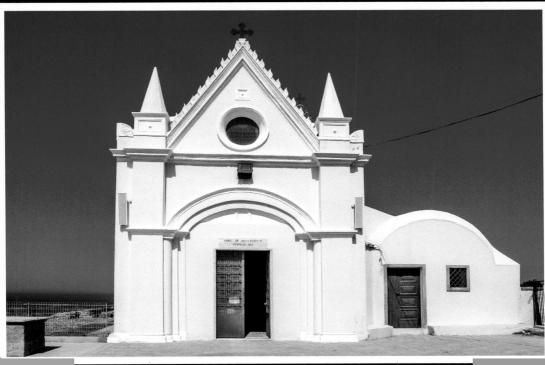

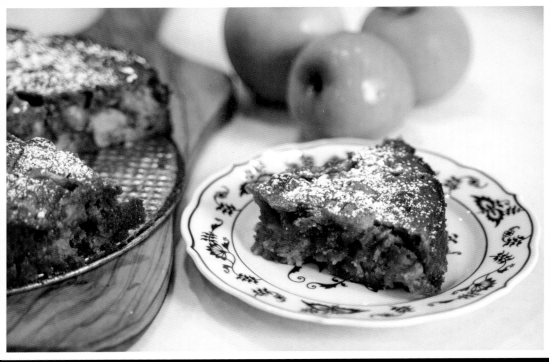

Apple, Almond, and Olive Oil Cake (Chapter 20)

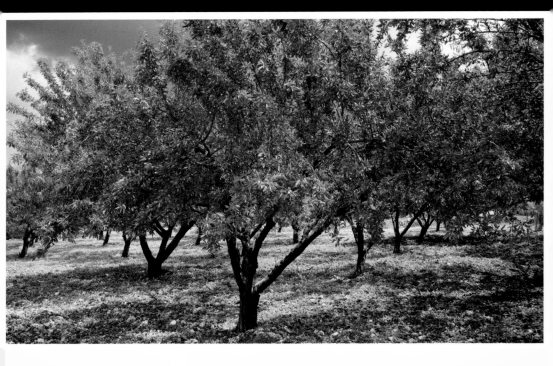

social activity, a cultural relic, and most of all, an important symbol of hospitality. Making the mental shift to valuing the preparation and enjoyment of natural, whole foods; getting regular physical activity; and making a commitment to enjoy foods in community whenever possible is important.

The following sections walk you through the pyramid from bottom to top and explain how to use it.

What each tier represents

The Mediterranean Diet Pyramid is made up of five tiers. Think of the bottom of the tier as the foundation — these are the things you should be doing most. And think of the top of the tier as the cherry on top — something to have once in a while, in small amounts.

Here are the five tiers of the pyramid, from bottom to top:

» **Be physically active. Enjoy meals with others.** This is the base of the pyramid, meaning that even before you think about what you eat, you should think about who you're going to eat with (see Chapter 5). Physical activity (see Chapter 7) is also critical to the Mediterranean way of life.

» **Fruits, vegetables, whole grains, olive oil, beans, nuts, legumes, seeds, herbs, and spices. Base every meal on these foods.** These are the foundation foods that you should center all your meals around.

» **Fish and seafood. Often, at least two times per week.** At least twice a week, you should eat a serving of fish or seafood.

» **Poultry, eggs, cheese, and yogurt. Moderate portions, daily to weekly.** You can find a wide range of quality when it comes to the foods in this category. Check out "Finding Daily Meal Examples from the Mediterranean," later in this chapter, for more information.

» **Meats and sweets. Less often.** These are special-occasion foods, traditionally eaten once a week and/or on holidays, depending upon the culture.

Off to the side of the pyramid, you see "Wine in moderation" and "Drink water." Wine and water are the traditional drinks of the Mediterranean diet — water is the main drink, and wine is enjoyed only in moderation. Countries in the Mediterranean region that don't have a local daily wine-drinking culture for religious regions — such as those in North Africa and some of the Middle Eastern countries in the region — do partake in antioxidant-rich tea and tisanes, as do wine-drinking countries.

Choosing water, green tea, or herbal tea over sugary drinks and alcohol offers many nutritional rewards. These drinks help to fill you up and keep your body hydrated. Green tea and herbal teas also offer a wide range of nutrients and have been shown to assist in weight loss. Depending on the type of herbal tea you choose, you can also enjoy other advantages. Ginger tea, for example has anti-inflammatory properties, helping to speed up digestion and calm the stomach. Dandelion tea assists the body with purifying the liver and promotes better digestion. Find out which teas suit your health goals, and enjoy them on a regular basis.

How to use the pyramid

The Mediterranean diet, like all other balanced diets, aims to meet basic nutritional needs by making sure that all the macronutrients (protein, fat, and carbohydrates) are present in each meal or snack. It also goes a few steps further to ensure you get healthful, nonprocessed, high-quality sources of protein (such as seafood, dairy, poultry, eggs, and meat on occasion), fat (such as nuts, olives, and extra-virgin olive oil), and carbohydrates (from unprocessed whole grains or vegetables such as potatoes and corn).

The first step to using the pyramid is to think about enjoying meals with others. Decide which meals you'll be able to eat in the company of other people. Chapter 3 offers some creative ways to do this, even for people who live alone. If you always eat alone, just adding one or two communal meals a week will pay off in the beginning!

Breaking bread or grabbing a bite with someone doesn't have to be reserved for romantic dates and family members. You can share a meal with work colleagues, your buddy from the softball team, or your best friend.

Plant-based foods make up the biggest portion of the pyramid, so the majority of your meals should be made up of these foods. Fruits, vegetables, whole grains, olive oil, beans, nuts, legumes, seeds, herbs, and spices should be the focus of every meal. You should be getting one or two servings of fresh vegetables at every meal. A single serving of whole grains, when served alongside protein and a healthful fat, will ensure that your macronutrient quotients are met. Fresh fruit should replace sugary confections for dessert and processed snacks. Nuts and seeds also make fantastic, portable snacks. A serving of legumes and beans will give you fiber, while extra-virgin olive oil, herbs, and spices provide flavor and health benefits.

In the plant-based foods section, you find what doctors now refer to as "eat-me-first foods" and "zero-calorie foods":

>> **Eat-me-first foods:** These include cruciferous vegetables such as broccoli, Brussels sprouts, cabbage, cauliflower, and kale. Combined with green leafy vegetables, extra-virgin olive oil, and nuts, these foods give you a lot of disease-preventing and health-boosting benefits.

>> **Zero-calorie foods:** These foods are said to burn more calories than they contain. Produce such as apples, arugula, asparagus, broccoli, cabbage, carrots, chard, cucumbers, grapefruit, and some lettuces fall in this category, so including servings of a few of them at meals is a great idea.

REMEMBER

Especially when discussing the plant-based portion of the pyramid, keep in mind that you should consume a wide *variety* of fruits and vegetables to get the most health benefits possible. "Eating the rainbow" is still good advice. Plus, our palates tend to get sick of eating the same thing over and over, so variety helps you to maintain a healthful eating style on a long-term basis.

Fish and seafood is the next tier up on the pyramid. Just one additional serving of fish or seafood per week can reduce your risk of heart disease by 49 percent, which explains why this tier is so important. Because most places in the Mediterranean region are near the Mediterranean Sea and/or other bodies of water, seafood was traditionally appreciated, prized, and plentiful. Choose varieties high in omega-3 fatty acids — such as mackerel, salmon, sardines, swordfish, and tuna — on a regular basis and supplement additional seafood for variety. Eating from this category two or more times a week is recommended.

The fourth tier of the pyramid is dedicated to poultry, eggs, cheese, and yogurt. You should eat moderate portions of these ingredients daily to weekly. If you're trying to lose weight, eat less of these foods. Even though they're a great source of protein, they can produce inflammation and oxidative stress in some people, especially if they aren't organic, so it's better to enjoy them in smaller quantities while you're trying to lose weight. When it comes to the Mediterranean lifestyle, quality is much more important than quantity in general, but when considering foods to add in from this tier, it's especially important to pay attention to the sources: Buy local, traceable, high-quality poultry, eggs, cheese, and yogurt.

Supermarkets do exist in the Mediterranean region, but most people still prefer to get their poultry and eggs from a local farm, farmers market, or butcher whom they trust (if they don't raise them on their own). Many Mediterranean countries still have strict quality regulations regarding cheese and yogurt. Often sold unpasteurized, people must consume the yogurt and other fresh (not aged) cheeses quickly, within a week.

MAKING SURE YOUR MEAL PLAN FITS YOUR NEEDS

One of the biggest advantages of the Mediterranean lifestyle is that it doesn't involve one uniform plan written in stone for everyone. Instead, it offers base guidelines — such as those found in the pyramid — and then allows the individual, the season, the culture, and the principle of pleasure to dictate how those guidelines are followed.

One of the forefathers of the Greek diet (which later became known as the Mediterranean diet) was Pythagoras. The legendary mathematician and philosopher founded a school in my ancestral hometown of Crotone, Italy (then known as Kroton), in the 6th century BCE when it was part of Magna Grecia. Pythagoras believed that humans should be vegetarian because he taught that we reincarnated as animals in other lives. In his school, which taught philosophy, music, and nutrition, in addition to mathematics, he forbade his students from eating meat or even plant-based foods that had a physiology similar to animal meat (such as fava beans). Despite Pythagoras's personal convictions, he allowed his son-in-law, the great Olympic champion Milo of Kroton, believed to be the strongest man in history, to eat meat. Pythagoras created a diet plan for Milo that included meat because his physical strength required it.

Your nutritional needs, health goals, personal preferences, and so on may differ from those of other people. For that reason, it's important to develop a plan that you enjoy and will be able to stick with, as well as one that will promote your health and happiness. The plan must also be doable within your own lifestyle, so it doesn't create unnecessary stress. In my own life, for example, I've seen that my mind, body, and spirit have had different requirements at different periods in time, so following one specific diet plan for my entire life doesn't make sense.

Sometimes we're more physically active, and we need more power. Other times, we're forced to be more sedentary or endure periods of challenges and stress. Maybe we're in the process of transforming an illness, pregnant with a baby, or adjusting to a new climate or job change. All these situations require special nutritional attention, different from those in our everyday lives.

If you need guidance in creating a meal plan (or several plans) that work well with your objectives, talk with a registered dietitian or nutritionist who believes in and promotes the Mediterranean lifestyle and can help you meet your objectives. If you start out with a plan like that, you don't have to do the same thing forever. Even people in the Mediterranean region who are having difficulty achieving the results that they want on their own or are responding to a particular health crisis consult professionals. These people can help clients get on track with what works well with their individual bodies and lifestyles.

Here are some daily eating guidelines to help you get started:

- Aim for 5 or 6 servings of fresh fruits and vegetables per day (with at least 4 being green leafy or cruciferous vegetables or bitter herbs). Eat the rainbow as much as possible when selecting produce.

- Eat 1 serving of beans or legumes per day.

- If you're a vegetarian, eat seeds and nuts to increase your protein intake.

- Consume 1 or 2 servings of good-quality dairy and/or poultry (eggs, yogurt, cheese, milk, chicken, or turkey) daily.

- Eat fish as your protein at least twice a week.

- Try to choose raw nuts, fresh fruits, fresh vegetables, or yogurt as a snack.

- Limit red meat and sweets to once a week or less.

- Make water and tisanes your top drink choices.

- Always have an idea of what to eat for the next meal.

Throughout history, people in the Mediterranean have relied on yogurt as a staple — and it can be a good one. In addition to cow milk, sheep and goat milk are usually used to make a wide variety of yogurts and cheeses in the region. These types of milk contain different nutrients and are believed to be higher in nutrients and easier to digest than the American varieties. Developing a palate for sheep and goat milk cheeses is a great way to get more nutrients and authentic Mediterranean flavor into your daily diet.

Last but not least, the top tier of the pyramid is devoted to meats and sweets. Although these two ingredients don't go together in a culinary sense, the point is that even normally "off-limits" foods are still permissible — as long as you don't consume them all the time. Plan to include high-fat and sugar-based desserts once a month and on holidays, for best results. New research even suggests that enjoying organic, lean meat more frequently, as part of a Mediterranean diet, isn't harmful.

Finding Daily Meal Examples from the Mediterranean

Mediterranean meal patterns differ greatly from those in the United States. And there isn't one particular meal plan that everyone in the region follows, so coming up with a formula that is effective yet authentic can be a struggle for newcomers to the lifestyle. All the countries in the Mediterranean enjoy breakfast, lunch, and dinner, but the way in which those meals are interpreted can vary greatly from country to country and region to region.

Breakfasts are probably the largest source of variance in the countries surrounding the Mediterranean basin. There is no one set way of doing breakfasts, so decide which breakfast works the best for you in terms of your likes and your lifestyle:

>> **If you love a large breakfast:** Take your cues from the Egyptians, Israelis, Lebanese, Moroccans, and Turks (to name a few), and enjoy a wide variety of items in the morning. In those countries, breakfasts usually consist of eggs, salads, a bean dish, fresh fruit, fresh cheeses, olives, yogurt, and fresh warm bread. That's just a base, though — some breakfasts can be much more elaborate than that! Most people take a single plateful of a bit of the aforementioned items and start their days with a full spectrum of nutrients. In the United States, this type of breakfast is especially suited to people who don't take lunches or eat much later in the day.

>> **If you prefer a light breakfast:** In places like the South of France, Italy, Portugal, and Spain, breakfast is much smaller and quicker, with some toast, marmalade, or a breakfast roll or fresh croissant and an espresso (often with milk). This light breakfast provides just enough energy to start the day, which leads up to a larger lunch. If you also eat a small lunch, this type of breakfast won't provide the amount of nutrients or calories that you'll need, so it probably won't be your best option.

REMEMBER

The common denominator among meals in the Mediterranean region is that, historically, lunches were the largest meal everywhere in terms of both quantity and types of foods. This way of eating stands in stark contrast to American meals, in which lunch is often smaller (or skipped) and eaten on the run. The benefit to having a larger and longer lunch is that you consume the majority of your calories during the part of the day when you're still able to convert those calories to energy and burn them off.

Deciding which type of breakfast to go with doesn't have to be static — you can have fun and change it up from day to day. For example, if you know that you'll be having a large lunch one day, you can start out with a lighter breakfast. If you know that lunch will come much later, or that you'll be doing intense physical activity, a heavier breakfast will be more beneficial to you. As an example, even though most Italians eat a very small breakfast made up of some type of pastry or biscotti and a quick coffee, Italian farmers traditionally enjoyed larger breakfasts — because their work was physically demanding, they often started their day with heavy staples such as sausage and polenta or frittatas.

Dinners, unless they're for entertaining purposes or special occasions, are usually lighter than lunches. In addition, they're often simpler and involve fewer intricate recipes.

The English word *supper* is derived from the French word *souper*, which meant dinner. The word *souper* was derived from the word *soup*, because dinners were often light. In modern times, the word *diner* is now used in France. In France, lunch is called *déjeuner* and breakfast is called *petit-déjeuner* ("little lunch"). Linguistically speaking, remembering these French terms can help you to eat the right things at the right time. A small "lunch" for breakfast, lunch being the main meal of the day, and a light dinner — perhaps a vegetable- and/or legume-based soup, an egg-based dish or fish, or a salad with some cheese and bread — can be great options that can be tailored to suit various seasons, palates, and culinary cultures within the Mediterranean region itself.

The following formulas are rough examples to use when you're making menus on your own:

>> **Breakfast:** 1 serving carbohydrate (usually from a whole-grain source), 1 serving protein (from beans, legumes, yogurt, or eggs), 1 serving healthy fat (olive oil or nuts), 1 serving fresh fruits and vegetables.

The carbohydrate usually comes from some type of bread, rusk, cookie, or toast. Good-quality plain Greek yogurt has the three macronutrients covered, so a bit of that with a serving of fruit or vegetables is enough to get your day off to a great start!

>> **Lunch:** 2 servings carbohydrate (usually from a whole-grain source), 1 serving protein, 1 serving healthy fat, 2 servings vegetables, and salad.

This would be the largest meal of the day, both in terms of quantity and types of foods served. Depending upon the country, the carbohydrate could be barley, couscous, pasta, rice, or wheat berries, as well as potatoes or starchy vegetables. The protein could be from beans, chicken, fish, legumes, or red meat. Vegetables could be served alone and/or incorporated into the carbohydrate and protein recipes, and some sort of fresh salad usually accompanies the meal.

>> **Dinner:** 1 serving carbohydrate (from a whole-grain source or a starchy vegetable), 1 serving protein, 1 serving healthy fat, 2 servings vegetables (usually 1 cooked and 1 green salad).

This meal, if eaten at home and served traditionally, could range from a soup or stew with bread and salad to a classically cooked protein with bread, a whole grain, or starchy vegetable, as well as a vegetable and salad.

Fresh fruit and nuts are served after meals (as desserts) or as snacks.

Reinventing Leftovers

Repurposing foods helps to stretch your time and your budget and literally enables you to get more out of the food that you make. Today you may hear this referred to as "leftover recycling" or adapting a "zero waste" food policy. People in the Mediterranean region and around the world have traditionally eaten leftovers because it was part of their lifestyle, not because it was trendy. Many sources will have you believe that this was done out of necessity, which is true. But before I talk about necessity, I need to introduce the concept of respect for food, ourselves, our land, our animals, our faith, and our communities.

People in the Mediterranean have traditionally made the most out of what they had out of respect. If Mother Nature provided you with a fennel plant, for example, why would you eat only the bulb and throw the rest away? In Southern Europe, fennel seeds, fennel bulbs, fennel stalks, and fennel fronds are prepared in many different ways. People can make everything from appetizers to desserts and liqueur by using various parts of the fennel plant.

Nowadays, we call this root-to-tip use of vegetables a novelty, but preparing food this way saves time and money while reducing waste and increasing well-being through the variety of foods that we eat. The nose-to-tail butchering used by trendy restaurants today is also nothing new. Years ago, meat was only eaten in the Mediterranean region for holidays, celebrations, and special occasions — not on a daily basis. When an animal was slaughtered or a fish was caught, it was used in its entirety out of respect for Mother Nature, our Creator, and the animal itself.

Waste was, and still is, seen as sacrilegious. A perfect example is the lamb that's eaten by Greeks as a part of the Orthodox Easter celebration. After the lamb is slaughtered, it's butchered in a way that enables people to cook it on a spit at Easter. The innards, instead of being thrown away, are transformed in to a mouthwatering soup called Marghiritsa, which is eaten after the midnight mass on Holy Saturday (the night before Easter). The lungs, liver, and heart make a savory broth and are then combined with eggs, rice, fresh herbs, lettuce, and parsley. The soup is the perfect antidote and celebratory meal after 40 days of veganism as a means of fasting during Lent. Leftover bits of lamb from Easter then get transformed into skillet gyro-type sandwich fillings, salad toppers, and wraps.

In Italy, the term *svuotafrigo* is what we may think of as "fridge foraging." Italians and other people in the region get really excited when they can turn their leftover tidbits taking up space in the fridge into a culinary masterpiece. Traditionally, there were two ways of fridge foraging:

» **Before a holiday and the New Year:** In Calabria, for example, there is a very popular, healthful, and nutritious soup recipe called *Millecosedde*. In dialect, this word means "a thousand little things" and it's like what Americans would call a minestrone — made up of leftovers from the fridge and pantry. This soup is made at New Year's so that people can start the New Year with new food and new energy. The Jewish tradition also promotes cleaning out the cupboards prior to Passover.

» **Before going shopping, on a set weekly or monthly basis:** As you start to run low on groceries, or know that you'll be shopping in a few days, you can make it a point to go through your pantry and fridge and make lists of what you've got left over. Then you can challenge yourself to prepare those foods in the best-tasting way possible. If you're new at this, the recipes in this book can provide you with a lot of inspiration. Or just search the web for what you've got on hand and the type of cuisine you want to make, and you'll find endless recipe suggestions.

REMEMBER

Leftovers are the ultimate way to make the most out of our food. Cooking a beautiful and nutritious meal is easy when you've got endless amounts of top shelf products and foods around you. When the variety is down to a minimum, however, that's when your creativity will be challenged!

Chapter **14**

Stocking a Mediterranean-Style Kitchen

P antries aren't just storage space for things that you purchase in bulk. Up until a century ago, kitchens all over the world required pantries in order to be able to provide balanced meals on a daily basis. Nowadays, a good pantry can set you up for cooking flavorful and nutritious meals in less time than it takes to order takeout.

In this chapter, I explain the Mediterranean approach to creating a pantry and show you how to tailor yours to your personal tastes and needs. I let you know which ingredients you need, as well as how to use them to create authentic Mediterranean meals without a recipe!

Filling Your Pantry with the Basics

A well-stocked pantry enables you to whip up a healthy, delicious meal any time. You'll never stand in your kitchen saying, "There's nothing to eat." When you have the right ingredients on hand, along with a strategy of when to use them, your pantry can become your best cooking partner!

In the following sections, I walk you through all the staple ingredients you should have in your pantry.

Cereals, pastas, and grains

Around the Mediterranean basin, *cereal* refers to specific types of grains, not the boxed, mass-produced, sugary breakfast cereals Americans are used to. Grains such as barley, buckwheat, cornmeal, farro, millet, oats, wheat berries, and whole-grain rice are the most common. Quinoa, wild rice, and other types rice are also popular, but they're recent additions. Bulgur, or cracked wheat, is popular in various sizes across the region.

In terms of pastas, couscous is the most popular in North Africa, while orzo and shorter noodles are eaten in Egypt, Greece, and Turkey. In the Levant, there is a larger couscous; known as "Israeli couscous" in the United States, in Lebanon it's known as *moghrabeya.* In Italy, there are thousands of types of dried pasta shapes and sizes.

When I buy packaged pasta, I always search for ones extruded in bronze dyes for their superior quality. Verrigni (https://verrigni.com) makes a product called Spaghettoro that is an artisan spaghetti extruded from gold dyes.

If gluten is a concern, look for gluten-free pasta options. A high-quality artisan pasta from Italy will tell you the type of wheat it's made from. Some companies use ancient grains such as farro, spelt, Senatore Capelli, and others to produce pastas that are much lower in gluten, even though they're made from wheat. Others add *superfoods* (foods that have a high concentration of nutrients), such as squid ink or spirulina (a form of algae), into their pastas for additional benefits.

WHAT'S OLD IS NEW AGAIN

The COVID-19 pandemic drove home the importance of a well-stocked pantry. Many people began paying attention to what they were buying and making sure they had enough on hand. But this experience still pales in comparison to the important role that pantries had in Mediterranean history. Before industrialization, and even much later in rural areas, there were no supermarkets in the Mediterranean.

Some people in the modern Mediterranean region have embraced supermarket shopping for its convenience and attractive prices, but many people still prefer to shop locally. There are communal, social, and health advantages to knowing the person you purchase your seafood, meats, vegetables, and baked goods from. For that reason, special (usually weekly) trips to the seafood mongers or marinas, butchers, produce markets, and bakeries are customary.

Originally a necessity and now an ideal lifestyle goal, many Mediterranean households prepared as many ingredients as they needed to at home and only supplemented with what they couldn't raise, grow, or trade themselves. This is still the way it's done on islands like Ikaria, Greece. In Southern Italy, where my family is from, the farming community prided themselves on only needing to buy olive oil, coffee, and sugar from outside sources. Those with olive trees only had to buy *two* ingredients from others!

Because restaurants were nonexistent (or not an option for families) throughout much of history, a pantry made the difference between eating complete meals and not. The cereals, pastas, grains, beans, legumes, nuts, seeds, and oils were what transformed garden-fresh produce and freshly caught fish, just harvested eggs, and fresh meat into the recipes and creations that we know today.

Before refrigerators and freezers, foods had to be pickled and preserved in order to be eaten out of season. Eating seasonally is best, but there are times when it's impossible. In the dead of winter, for example, during a blizzard, there isn't much fresh produce to be had. In addition, some crops have really short growing seasons. If a variety of bean, such as the cranberry bean, for example, is only grown for a week or two per year, and it's your favorite bean, preserving it to enjoy throughout the year is a great idea. Some vegetables have such huge bumper crops (think zucchini, eggplant, and tomatoes at the end of the summer) that it's impossible to eat them all at once. Instead of wasting those foods, wise people preserved them in a variety of ways to be enjoyed throughout the year.

Rice varies from place to place in the Mediterranean. Spain is known for its Bomba rice and Calasparra rice, which are used to make paellas and other dishes. Italy boasts the Arborio, Carnaroli, and Vialone Nano varieties for risotto, salads, and more. Egypt has its own rice known as "Egyptian rice" in Middle Eastern markets; it's similar to the Spanish rice and Italian rice because it was brought to Europe in the 9th century from Egypt. In Turkey, the same short, starchy type of rice is called baldo rice. Moroccans have traditionally used short-grain rice, but basmati rice is gaining in popularity across the region. Long-grain rice is usually preferred in the Levant portion of the Mediterranean.

For best results, set your pantry up with the following:

>> A variety of the whole grains that you like the most

>> Pasta shapes and types that you like

>> Varieties of rice that compliment your style of cooking

>> Products that cook in minutes, such as fine bulgur wheat, oats, and quinoa

If you like a variety of cooking styles and the various styles of cooking in the Mediterranean, stock up on as many of these types of products as possible. When you need a nutritious meal in a pinch, you can find culinary inspiration and nutritional foundations in this category. Main dishes, side dishes, breakfasts, snacks, and puddings can all be made from these ingredients.

Beans and legumes

Beans and legumes were a main protein staple throughout history in the Mediterranean region. No matter which Mediterranean country you go to today, you'll find endless ways to prepare them. At least one meal per day in the Mediterranean region usually contains 1 serving (½ cup cooked) of beans or lentils. The pantry is the perfect place to store them.

When it comes to beans and legumes, dried varieties are your best bets in terms of cost and sodium content. That said, it's a good idea to keep some canned beans and chickpeas on hand for when you don't have time to soak them in advance.

The most popular beans and legumes in the Mediterranean region are broad beans, cannellini beans, chickpeas, cranberry beans (also called Roman or borlotti beans), fava beans, flageolet beans, navy beans, and yellow split peas. Red, green, brown, and black lentils are all also popular. There are so many good varieties available on the market that there is no need to look for specific brands or types. It can be fun, however, to search out French Puy lentils, heirloom varieties from Italy, or even those from your local farmers market.

PROTECTING QUALITY

Biodiversity is highly prized in the Mediterranean region. and beans are the type of crops that are usually grown in between peak seasons of a farm or estate's main industry. Many of the winegrowers I know plant beans in the fields after the annual grape harvest, for example. This helps to enrich the soil and makes better use of the land. Beans and legumes are easy on the environment. Many cities and towns in the region are known for their owns specific varieties of beans and lentils, and they market them as special Protected Documentation of Origin products. (This designation was implemented by the European Union to protect product names from misuse and imitation and assist consumers by giving them information concerning the specific character of products.) There is a trend, especially in the European portion of the Mediterranean, to reintroduce the growing of ancient and heirloom beans, grains, grapes, and olives.

The new interest in ingredients that have often been taken for granted has helped to make these healthful and historic foods grow in popularity. Their fiber and protein content makes them a good addition to the diet of those who are trying to build muscle. Because of their carbohydrate content, however, people trying to lose weight should limit their intake to one serving per day.

TIP

To prepare the beans for cooking, just place the amount you would like to cook in a large bowl and cover them with water. Place a plate or lid on the top and allow them to soak and cook. Then, depending on the type of bean, you can cook them by simmering them in water or broth until they're tender, about 1 hour. I like to cook enough beans to last me all week. That way, I can store them in the refrigerator and add them to soups, sauces, salads, or rice pilafs when I need them.

TIP

To cook lentils, just rinse them in cold water and sort them with your fingers to make sure that there are no small stones in the mix. (In the United States, I've only had this happen once, but overseas, it's much more common, so I always sort them well for good measure.) Then cook them in the same fashion as you would cook beans, until tender. (Lentils do not require soaking before cooking.) Note that red lentils cook up in just a few minutes, while green and brown lentils could take 30 to 40 minutes depending upon their variety. Small black lentils and other varieties take much longer to cook.

Extra-virgin olive oil

In Italian, there is a saying, *Olio nuovo, vino vecchio*, that means "New oil, old, wine." It's important to keep that phrase in mind when you're adding oil to your pantry — you don't want to keep anything around from longer than the previous year's harvest.

If you keep extra-virgin olive oil in a cool, dark, place it *could* stay safe for a few years. It takes a while for it to go rancid, normally. But just because it isn't rancid doesn't mean you want to consume it. The older the oil gets, the more nutrients it loses, so it may taste great, but it won't be as good for you.

Olive harvests generally take place from late October to November in most places in the Mediterranean. By the time the production process is finished and they're ready to be exported to the United States, it could be a few weeks, so that would be December. Then it takes a while for the container to arrive in the United States, for the product to be shipped to the stores, and for it to be put on store shelves. Best-case scenario, it's usually January before you can get our hands on the latest harvest's oil.

When you buy a commercial extra-virgin olive oil at the store, don't just look for the expiration date — look for the pressed-on date. If it doesn't have one, make sure you're purchasing something that is far away from the expiration date because sometimes those are up to three years after the actual pressing of the olives.

To enhance the flavor and dining experience, instead of using an all-purpose olive oil, pair each dish with the olive oil that's best suited to it. Just as you pair wine with certain dishes, you can pair olive oil with certain dishes. Experiment with different varieties using different types of olives from different countries to see what you like best. In addition to my own privately labeled olive oil (Amy Riolo Selections), which is a blend of three Italian cultivars — Gentile di Chieti, Intosso, and Leccino — I also keep Tierra Callada's Spanish Picual on hand for spicier dishes and Alessandro Anfosso's Taggiasca extra-virgin olive oil, which has a buttery flavor and is perfectly suited to baked goods and mashed potatoes. I also love Greek Koroneiki olive oil, which I use for my authentic Greek dishes.

In addition to its great flavor, *honest* olive oil (produced by single estates that are completely traceable and use the best practices) provides such amazing health benefits that the claims are too many to list. Because olive oil is one of the ingredients that's enjoyed throughout the entire Mediterranean region, and it's available abroad and easy to study, researchers use it to determine the efficacy of the Mediterranean diet.

Because of its anti-inflammatory benefits, extra-virgin olive oil is good for reducing the root cause of all illness: inflammation. With natural blood-thinning benefits, it does everything from prevent the formation of blood clots and lower the level of total blood cholesterol to reduce the risk of breast cancer and colon cancer. These are just a few of the many benefits of extra-virgin olive oil.

TIP

The term *extra-virgin* is about acidity. By definition, extra-virgin olive oil has to have an acidity rate of 0.8 or less. The lower the acidity rate, the higher the quality. Italian olive oil quality is denoted by the following geographic indicators (strictly enforced government regulations on the quality of products that come from specific geographic areas):

» **Varieties:** There are more than 1,200 varieties of olives. Increasingly, many smaller producers are offering single-variety olive oils so consumers can become familiar with a particular type. Different varieties have different colors and flavors, which makes them perfectly suited for pairing with different foods. Just like wine, each olive has different notes that play off the foods that they're paired with.

» **Polyphenols:** Polyphenols are antioxidants present in some natural foods such as extra-virgin olive oil, red wine, and dark chocolate. The variety of olive(s) in an oil determine its overall polyphenol level. The antioxidant properties of polyphenols have been widely studied, and they're known to assist in the prevention of degenerative diseases.

You can discover the strength of the polyphenols in an olive oil at home by taking a sip and then slurping it back. As you make the slurping noise, the oil will coat your throat. After a few minutes, you should feel a burn. The stronger the burn, the higher the amount of polyphenols in the oil.

Single-estate producers usually post their polyphenol levels on their websites. Different cultivars naturally have different levels of polyphenols, and each year's harvest will yield slightly different results.

» **Cold pressing:** Extra-virgin olive oil should normally be made using a process called *cold pressing*. *Cold* means that the olives have been kept no higher than 81.9 degrees, and *pressing* refers to the method of extraction. In cold pressing, no heat or chemical additives are used to extract the oil from the olives (heat and chemical additives can alter and destroy the flavors and aromas of the olive oil). This way, the olive oil retains its full nutritional value.

Putting *cold pressed* on a label isn't really necessary because it's standard. *First cold-pressed* means that the olive juice was obtained from literally the first pressing of the olives. It the olden days, this was a big deal because those olives offered the most nutritional value. Nowadays, it doesn't mean anything because the olives are put in centrifuges to extract the oil.

» **Filtration:** Many purists prefer the flavor and quality of unfiltered olive oil, but some people are turned off by the sediment found at the bottom of bottles of unfiltered oil. For this reason, many farmers are using a natural filtration method that involves placing the oil in cisterns and switching it from tank to tank once a month, allowing the sediment to filter out naturally. This time-consuming process, maintains the integrity of the oil without the undesired sediment.

TIP

Like everything else, if you want to be sure that you're consuming the best-quality olive oil, try to look for bottles where the producer is most traceable. Single-estate varieties, for example, can be traced right back to the source, and you'll know exactly what you're getting.

Condiments and flavor enhancers

This is where vinegars, mustards, tomato pastes, capers, anchovy fillets, salts, and spices come into play. You can really add a lot of flavor to your cooking by keeping these items on hand. Condiment preferences vary from country to country.

TIP

Have a high-quality, aged balsamic vinegar on hand for drizzling, as well as a younger one for vinaigrettes. White, distilled vinegar; red and white wine vinegars; and other specialty vinegars also add flavor and health benefits to your meals.

My Amy Riolo Selections Vinegar is imported from the famous Castelli vinegar makers in Italy and is made from 100 percent Trebbiano grapes in a similar process to the way that balsamic vinegar is made, except that the single white variety of grape produces a balsamic flavor yet is completely transparent instead of brown. It adds a natural sweetness and excellent mouthfeel to recipes.

In terms of herbs, spices, and seeds, I keep on hand those that are found in the Mediterranean region and will provide me with improved health and enhanced flavor, including the following:

>> Allspice

>> Anise seeds

>> Caraway seeds

>> Cayenne

>> Cinnamon (the pure, Ceylon variety)

>> Cloves (ground and whole)

>> Coriander (ground)

>> Cumin (ground)

>> Fennel seeds

>> Flaxseeds

>> Ginger (ground)

>> Green cardamom pods

- Herbes de Provence
- Marjoram
- Mint (dried)
- Nutmeg (whole)
- Oregano
- Paprika
- Peppercorns
- Red pepper (crushed)
- Saffron
- Sage
- Sea salt (unrefined)
- Sesame seeds
- Sumac
- Tarragon
- Thyme
- Turmeric
- Za'atar

Baking ingredients

In order to be able to whip up your own wholesome baked goods when the mood strikes, be sure to keep the following on hand:

- Active dry yeast
- Almond milk (or another shelf-stable milk)
- Baking powder
- Baking soda
- Cocoa powder (fair trade, unsweetened)
- Cornmeal
- Cornstarch

>> Flours (almond, unbleached all-purpose, barley, chickpea, semolina, whole wheat)

>> Polenta

>> Sugar (natural)

>> Vanilla extract

Nuts and dried fruits are an important part of the Mediterranean diet and should be kept in the pantry. Often served alone as a snack or dessert, they're also usually the protagonists of sweet recipes or used as a garnish for rice dishes. I recommend keeping the following in your pantry:

>> Almonds

>> Chestnuts

>> Dates

>> Pine nuts

>> Pistachios

>> Raisins

>> Walnuts

Combined with fresh fruit and nuts, these staples can produce impressive desserts and breads rather quickly.

Honey is an important element in the Mediterranean diet. Throughout the region, local honey made from a wide variety of flowers and plants is used. Honeys are coveted for their delicious taste, health benefits, and curative properties. Chestnut, eucalyptus, lavender, oregano, wild thyme, wildflower, and scores of other honeys are indigenous to the reason. I like to keep eucalyptus honey from Calabria, wild thyme honey from Ikaria, and chestnut honey from Abruzzo in my pantry, along with goldenrod honey, which is local to the region of the United States where I live.

TIP

Many healthcare professionals believe that by eating honey made from local plants, especially those that are the sources of seasonal allergies, can help people to combat them. Honeys last for a long time and taste great stirred into tisanes, drizzled on fresh fruit or desserts, and eaten on their own as a health-boosting tonic.

Few Mediterranean pantries are void of coffees, teas, and tisanes. Regional tastes vary, but usually at least one of these will be found in everyone's cupboard:

» **Coffees:** Recent studies claim that boiled coffees, such as the varieties that are consumed in Egypt, Greece, Turkey, and the Levant are high in polyphenols and antioxidants. Because they contain only a moderate amount of caffeine, they're good for your heart and relatively better than other coffee beverages.

» **Teas:** Both black and green teas are enjoyed in the Mediterranean. In Morocco, green tea with mint is the drink of choice, while most other Mediterranean countries enjoy varieties of black tea (unless they're on a diet, when green tea is favored). Black tea is grown in Turkey, where there is a long-standing tradition of tea drinking and tea rooms. In Egypt, black tea is also widely consumed.

» **Tisanes:** Tisanes are hot, tea-style drinks made out of herbs and spices. In the Mediterranean region, several styles of tisanes are available, each touted for its health benefits and drunk for certain reasons. You may be familiar with chamomile for sleeping, but anise is also used for colds, ginger for upset stomachs, wild thyme for respiratory issues, oregano as an immune booster, hibiscus for lowering blood pressure, dandelion root and milk thistle for detoxifying the liver, and so on. A delicious apple tisane is also a favorite drink in Turkey. One of my favorite tisanes in Egypt is made out of cinnamon with water or hot milk. The cinnamon has anti-inflammatory and blood-sugar-leveling benefits, and the smell is divine.

Tisanes can be purchased in boxes with individual bags and stored in the pantry or made out of the spices. To make a tisane with a tea bag, steep the bag in hot water, covered, for 10 minutes; remove the bag; and drink. To make a tisane with loose spices, steep in hot water, covered, for 10 minutes; then strain the tea into another cup and enjoy. Most people drink tisanes before bed, after meals, or when they aren't feeling well.

Canned and jarred goods

You won't find too many canned goods in Mediterranean kitchens. Most of the items that people preserve themselves are called "canned" even though they usually store them in glass jars. In addition to items that people can themselves, fruit preserves and marmalades, canned or jarred fish (such as anchovies, mackerel, salmon, sardines, and tuna) are common pantry items. Dried porcini mushrooms or other types of mushrooms in oil or vinegar are good to store in the pantry as well. Vegetables that don't need to be refrigerated (such as potatoes, onions, garlic, and shallots) are usually stored in pantries, too.

For flavor and health benefits, a wide variety of pickles are consumed in the Mediterranean. Everything from the Italian vegetable Giardiniera to Moroccan preserved lemons and an Egyptian combination of the two are common. People store chili pepper pastes, jars of vegetables and fruits, and more. I recommend jarred artichokes, olives, and roasted red peppers. Jarred tomato purees and whole tomatoes are essential for sauces, stews, and soups. Keep jarred tahini (sesame puree) on hand to make hummus and baba ghanouj. In addition, plain breadcrumbs, whether homemade or store-bought, are good to have on hand. A handful of any of these ingredients will turn a bland meal into a Mediterranean celebration of flavors!

Filling Your Fridge and Freezer

Nothing beats fresh food, and stocking a few of the right ingredients can help you take your pantry items to new heights. I also like to call the freezer the modern American pantry because people in the United States are typically much more comfortable using their freezers than people in the Mediterranean region are.

Fresh foods to have on hand

Because plants are the foundation of the Mediterranean diet and fresh fruits and vegetables are what you're supposed to be eating the most of, it's a good idea to have them ready to eat. Try to have all the colors of the rainbow represented in your refrigerator. You can't go wrong with fresh cruciferous vegetables and leafy greens in terms of nutrients, so try to stock several varieties of the ones you like the most.

In terms of protein sources, meat, seafood, and dairy are all part of the traditional Mediterranean diet and should be kept in stock unless you're a vegan or allergic to them. Choose the best-quality local milk, eggs, and cheeses that you can find. Full-fat Greek yogurt (especially those made of sheep and goat milk if you can find them) are full of probiotics, inulin, and macronutrients. Low-fat cheeses, such as mozzarella, ricotta, and cottage cheese, as well as a variety of aged cheeses from cow, sheep, and goat sources, add a lot of flavors, vitamins, and minerals to meals.

The freezer: The modern pantry

Many professional chefs freak out when I use the word *freezer*. Fresh is always preferred over frozen, but that doesn't make frozen foods the enemy. Because some vegetables are frozen at their peak, frozen versions can actually be *better* than produce that's stored for months and shipped from around the globe. In addition, if making a dinner out of frozen fish and vegetables prevents you from calling for delivery or takeout, you're doing your wallet and your waistline a favor.

Here's what I like to keep on hand in my freezer:

>> Berries

>> Fish

>> Meat (beef, chicken, veal, and so on)

>> Vegetables

>> Whole-wheat pita and other breads

>> Extra portions of what I cook and bake

When I bake, I always make at least double the recipe and freeze the extra. This way, when I'm short on time, I can always enjoy something fresh and homemade instead of having to buy it. I use the same technique for cooking. Sauces, soups, stews, and stocks freeze well. I make extra and store the remainder in portion-size plastic containers. On days when I know that I won't have time to cook, I can defrost them and enjoy homemade food.

Pantry Cooking Formulas for Quick Meals

You can put well-stocked pantries to good use in numerous ways. Keep this list nearby so you can whip up a tasty and nutritious meal any time:

>> **Bean dip:** Beans; spices; extra-virgin olive oil

>> **Bean, lentil, and vegetable skillet:** Beans; lentils; vegetables; extra-virgin olive oil; spices

>> **Bean soup:** Beans; stock; tomato puree; extra-virgin olive oil

>> **Bean stew:** Beans; stock; tomato puree; spices

>> **Beans or lentils and rice:** Lentils and/or beans; rice; caramelized onions or chili paste

>> **Chickpea or bean salad:** Chickpeas or beans; extra-virgin olive oil; vegetables; spices

>> **Cooked wheat, barley, or bulgur cereal:** Cooked grain; milk; dried fruits and nuts; honey or sugar

>> **Date, almond, and sesame balls:** Dates; almonds; sesame seeds

>> **Falafel:** Chickpeas; spices; extra-virgin olive oil; garlic; onions; tahina

>> **Hummus:** Chickpeas; tahini; extra-virgin olive oil

>> **Lentil dip:** Lentils; stock; spices

>> **Lentil soup:** Lentils; stock; tomato puree; extra-virgin olive oil; vegetables

>> *Minestre* **(minestrone-style soup):** Pasta (or other grain); beans; stock; tomato puree; extra-virgin olive oil; vegetables

>> **Pasta and beans:** Pasta; beans; stock; tomato puree; extra-virgin olive oil

>> **Pasta salad:** Pasta; vegetables; extra-virgin olive oil

>> **Pasta with fish:** Pasta; tuna (or other fish); extra-virgin olive oil; olives and/or tomato sauce

>> **Pasta with tomato sauce and vegetables:** Pasta; garlic; extra-virgin olive oil; chili paste; tomato puree

>> **Rice pilaf:** Basmati rice; vegetable, beans, or legumes; toasted nuts; dried fruit

>> **Rice pudding:** Rice; milk; dried fruits and nuts; honey or sugar

>> **Rice salad:** Rice; olives; extra-virgin olive oil; canned vegetables; beans

>> **Roasted chickpeas:** Chickpeas; spices; extra-virgin olive oil

>> **Semolina or wheat pudding:** Semolina or wheat; honey; dried fruit; milk

>> **Spaghetti with garlic, oil, and chilies:** Spaghetti; extra-virgin olive oil; chili paste; garlic

>> **Tuna salad:** Tuna; extra-virgin olive oil; vegetables

>> **Wheat, barley, or bulgur soup:** Cooked grain; stock; beans or legumes

>> **Vegetable couscous:** Couscous; stock; vegetables; spices; extra-virgin olive oil

These items can be made strictly from the pantry alone. When you add in fresh and frozen ingredients, the sky is the limit in terms of taste and creativity!

REMEMBER

It takes a little time to set up a pantry in the beginning, but the rewards are extremely worthwhile.

Chapter **15**

Shopping for Food the Mediterranean Way

I n the modern world, shopping is often seen as a chore. But there is no reason to view it this way. Traditionally, procuring food was one of the greatest pleasures in life. In this chapter, I show you fun ways of getting the most out of your shopping and eating experience.

Bringing the Fun Back to Shopping for Food

So many people in the United States *love* shopping for jewelry, clothes, cars, boats, bikes, and electronics, but they view grocery shopping as a chore. When I was growing up, shopping and procuring food was one of our greatest joys. Even though we weren't farmers, we grew many things, and my grandfather taught me the pleasures of "getting the best" ingredients you could, even if you bought them.

Living through different types of adversity — whether lack of food, money, or choices — definitely makes you appreciate the little things more. Older civilizations have faced so many more problems than our modern societies have — it's only natural that they derive more happiness from the simple task of being picky about what they eat.

Nowadays, even though we have all the choices and possibilities in the world, we've lost appreciation for the bounties of nature. Getting back in touch with your sense of gratitude for the mere ability to choose what you want will benefit your cooking and your health as well.

TIP

If you aren't in the habit of shopping for your own food or you don't enjoy it, come up with a simple strategy to make it more pleasurable. The ability to "sing in the rain" and find ways to enjoy the mundane is, after all, one of the fundamental concepts of the Mediterranean lifestyle.

Letting inspiration be your guide

At the beginning of each season, I like to take a trip to local farms that have stands or shops set up on their property. It's a fun outing, and some places even let you pick your own fruits and vegetables. I see a lot of American families visiting the farms during pumpkin season in anticipation of Halloween, but not much beyond that. I guarantee you that the little hands in your family will have just as much fun if you let them make figures and faces out of broccoli and other vegetables!

If you grow your own food, you know the difference in taste between something homegrown versus something store-bought. All produce is that way. Even a humble potato or head of broccoli will taste vastly different if you purchase it at a farm or a farmers market or grow it yourself. I really look forward to the fresh fall broccoli that has much more flavor and nutrients than store-bought varieties. Even though I don't go to the farms weekly, a seasonal trip allows me to stock up on great vegetables and get inspired for the season ahead. It gives me a good idea of what's available, and I get additional inspiration to plan my menus that way.

It's easy to become accustomed to hearing what you *shouldn't* eat. When tasked with shopping, you may be stuck. Maybe you're trying to cut down on sugar or carbs or shopping for a family member with an allergy — or all three! Perhaps you've just read three different news reports that said foods you thought were healthful were actually bad for you. When this happens, it's only natural that shopping for food loses its appeal.

I say it's time to take back the reins of control and make the best out of the situation. Historically, people didn't even have the luxury of giving up an ingredient by choice. They couldn't afford sugar because it was too expensive, there were prohibitive taxes on wheat and salt, and perhaps the crop of a season was much less than what was anticipated. Nowadays, worst-case scenario, one store may not have something, but you can still go to another. With the exception of a few luxury ingredients, staple foods are regularly inexpensive in the United States.

With that in mind, you can be thankful for the choices you have, what you can eat, and the ability to shop. Then you can get inspired by the foods you want to experience more of. I like to call the process of daydreaming about food "culinary guided imagery." A little goes a long way.

The following list will get your creative culinary juices flowing:

1. **Write down a list of all the foods that you and the people you're shopping for *can* eat.**

   Separate it into categories like fruits, vegetables, protein, dairy, beans and legumes, and so on.

2. **Go over your list and circle the foods you and your family *like* to eat the most.**

3. **Underline the foods that are nutritional staples and that you need to have on hand (especially if you didn't circle them in Step 2).**

4. **Spend a few minutes thinking about the best versions of the foods you circled that you've ever tasted and write those down.**

For example, maybe your list had sweet potatoes circled and you remember an oven-roasted version that you loved. Or maybe broccoli makes you remember a soup that your mother used to make. When I see kale, I think of my grandmother's kale and potatoes, which she made during Lent on Fridays because we couldn't eat meat — even though it was a simple dish, it brings back happy memories.

If you ponder each food on your list this way and write down some inspiration for each one, you'll be well on your way to getting back into the swing of things. When you've exhausted everything you can think of, try thinking about restaurant meals and include those, too. Then look to TV shows, websites, magazines, and cookbooks for inspiration. Pick up your favorite cookbook and browse through the index for some of the ingredients on your list. You'll come up with even more ways to enjoy those foods!

When you have several entries for each food on your list of inspiration, type it up or save it on your phone. Your goal is to come up with enough meal ideas to feed yourself and those you cook for until the next time you go shopping. So, if you shop once a week, you need 7 breakfasts, 7 lunches, 7 dinners, and 14 snacks — multiplied by the number of people you need to feed. If you put all that together, and then go to make a list, it can be a bit overwhelming, so I create separate sections of my list, which I then separate into different stores or sections of the same store. This saves times and is a lot more organized.

Looking for fun in all the right places

Even if you never leave your home, you can enjoy a rich and varied diet, just by ordering groceries delivered to your door. This option is an important and valuable one for many people, and one that I took advantage of during the COVID-19 pandemic. Still, I couldn't wait to have the opportunity to go to the store to choose ingredients on my own. People in the Mediterranean region, given the choice, always choose to shop where they can see and touch the food prior to buying it.

In addition to making sure you're getting good-quality foods, if you shop for ingredients yourself, you enjoy a connection to the food that has a psychological reward. Just looking at food, smelling it, and touching it helps you to eat less and digest your food better. Plus, it's just plain fun!

Part of being a good cook is knowing how to pair ingredients together. Without smelling them, or knowing what they smell like, that's difficult to do. In most cases, smelling foods is the best way of determining their freshness and ripeness. For example, if fresh fruit doesn't have a smell, it's probably not ripe yet. On the other hand, if fish smells "fishy," it's past its prime — fresh fish smells like the ocean.

Shopping yourself also gives you the advantage of being able to eye the food. If something is old or moldy, you won't buy it, but it might make it into your bags if you're ordering your groceries online. Picking out the right food — and getting the most for your money — is part of the fun of shopping.

Another great reason to love shopping is that it gives you inspiration. People in the Mediterranean region always start out with a list of what they need — but when they get to the market and see a bright, beautiful, just harvested pile of artichokes or dandelion greens, they'll add them to the cart as well. When you shop for your own food, those simple pleasures don't have to be reserved for a week or two of the year — they can be each week or each time you go shopping.

TIP

Farmers markets, supermarkets, international grocery stores, and CSA boxes are fantastic ways to get the most out of shopping. I always suggest mixing it up to not only get the most out of your budget but also make it more fun. Mental health experts even suggest changing or alternating supermarkets as a way of keeping your mind healthy. Sometimes if you shop at the same place for too long, it not only gets boring but also helps to reinforce any negative habits that we may have.

If you have a farmers market in your area, I highly recommend visiting it. You'll form beautiful friendships with people in the community, purchase better ingredients, eat seasonally, and support the environment and local business all in one stop. I have never visited a farmers market without leaving feeling happier and more inspired. Sometimes you'll find things that you don't "need" but that you couldn't wait to eat. Other times, you'll find plants and foods that seemed to have disappeared from markets but that you remember eating as a child (such as Italian prune plums, teeny eggplants, and cranberry beans, in my case). The dairy products found at most farmers markets are a revelation in taste, freshness, and good agricultural practices.

Supermarkets get a bad rap, but there is no need to bash them. Large businesses need to respond to demand to stay afloat, and our purchasing power determines what they stock on their shelves. If you want to get the most out of your local store, stay on the outer perimeter of the store while shopping. In many U.S. supermarkets, the stuff that's good for you — such as produce, dairy, meats, and seafoods — are usually kept in those areas. If you want to reap the rewards of the Mediterranean lifestyle, packaged foods are not your priority. Patronize supermarkets for their convenience and great assortment of products, but try your best to purchase the types of foods that would have been available in your great-grandparents' time.

I love international supermarkets because they normally stock a lot of wonderful pantry items and produce that you simply can't get anywhere else. I recommend going to one international market at least once a month or stocking up every few months, so you can get great deals on fresh and diverse items that you wouldn't find elsewhere. If you're making a lot of Mediterranean-inspired dishes, go to Greek, Italian, Middle Eastern, North African, Spanish, and other markets — they have a much larger array of those types of ingredients. Luckily, many of these specialty ingredients can be found in traditional supermarkets, too, but exploring different places will give you more inspiration and help to stretch your budget, as well as increase your choices.

A traditional supermarket, for example, may offer you one or two choices of tahini paste or orange blossom water, while a Middle Eastern market will give you closer to ten. In my area, even the larger Korean and Indian supermarkets carry a wider amount of fresh fruits and vegetables, seafood, and Mediterranean pantry ingredients than traditional supermarkets do, so I often recommend shopping at them as well.

CSA boxes are another great way to "shop" and incorporate more seasonal and local produce into your diet. These programs work with a specific farm or an entire network of farms to provide customers freshly picked produce delivered to their doors. What I love the most about CSA boxes is that they're a modern way to eat Mediterranean. Getting that box of ingredients really teaches you what's seasonal in your area. Sometimes you get more of a specific vegetable (such as turnips or *ramps* [wild onions that grow in the Eastern portion of North America in the spring], for example) than you may want. But, just like people in Casablanca, Constantinople, Cyprus, Jerusalem, and Provence did since the beginning of time, you have to think of creative ways to use them. If you sign up for a CSA and really get into the process, you'll find that it improves your cooking, your health, and your community.

Making a List, Checking It Twice

Taking the time to make a list of what you need and want, for all the meals and snacks you'll be preparing between the time you go shopping and your next shopping trip will have big payoffs.

Everyone is busy, and getting creative with your shopping list can seem trivial when there are more important things to take care of in your life. The extra time it takes to make a good list, however, can save you time, energy, and money, and improve your health, while putting better food on the table, so it's well worth the investment.

Whether I'm making my shopping list for a cooking class, a large corporate event, or myself, I always use the same Mediterranean strategy. Traditionally, in the countries around the Mediterranean basin, people shopped at several different stores. When I'm in Egypt, Greece, Italy, Morocco, and Turkey today, we shop for seafood at the fish monger or marina, bread at the bakery, fruits and vegetables at the produce market, meats at the butcher, and dairy products at the farm or vendor. Weekly shopping is usually supplemented with foraging by someone in the family. Often, there will be a particular family member — maybe a parent, an aunt or uncle, or a grandparent — who heads to the fields or nearby mountains or other outside area to pick nature's bounty, such as wild asparagus, mushrooms. berries, fresh herbs, and so on. In more rural areas, picking your own produce and foraging with the family starts first. Whatever you can't get that way is bought.

TIP

Make a list of what's in your pantry and subtract or add to it as necessary. That way, you'll always know what you have on hand. I recommend also keeping a copy of the Mediterranean Diet Pyramid on your fridge and close by whenever you're making shopping lists and weekly meal plans. Eventually, it'll become second nature.

When you get the hang of planning out your own meals, as well as the chance to eat and enjoy them, you'll be impressed by the quality and quantity of foods you can prepare for yourself, as well as how good they make you feel. Chapter 16 gives some authentic inspiration for what to make and when.

TIP

Any Mediterranean shopping list should have the following sections:

- » Produce
- » Pantry
- » Seafood
- » Dairy
- » Meat
- » Bread/bakery
- » Household (nonfood) items

Separating the list like this will save time if you go to one grocery store so you don't have to keep track of what's where. If you like to go to different stores and also take advantage of the farmers market, for example, you could take the produce and the dairy section there, while you get your pantry items from the international market, meat from a butcher, and baked goods from a bakery. Sometimes the farmers markets will carry everything except for the pantry and household items.

Practical tips for meal planning

Part of the success of a good list is the meal planning that took place before writing it. If there is no meal planning, a list is simply the ingredients that are missing from your house or that you think you'll need. If you plan meals and snacks ahead of time, and incorporate those ingredients into your list, it'll be much more effective. Plus, it'll save you from going back to the store, ordering takeout, and making poor food choices.

TIP

Pull out a large calendar that you can write on or get a notebook and a pen. Note which days you'll have more, less, or no time to cook based on your other activities. Honestly evaluate which items you and those you eat with would like to eat when (for example, if Wednesday nights are always busy, simpler meals or ones you can make in advance may be best). Fill in breakfast, lunch, snacks, and dinner for every day.

Now, look at the meals that you want to eat and when. Go back through each recipe and add to your shopping list the ingredients that you need.

If you feel intimidated by this process, know that you aren't alone. If there are places where you enjoy shopping located close to you, you may want to make more frequent trips in order to not have to prep and plan so much in advance. As long as you know what you need before you get to the store, you can make sure to have all your bases covered. And have fun supplementing with "new" and interesting items you find along the way!

5 Authentic Mediterranean Recipes for All Occasions

Get to the core of what the healthful Mediterranean cultures have traditionally eaten and when.

Discover why breakfast matters and become familiar with distinct styles of eating in the morning across the region.

Embrace the scores of dazzling small plates that precede many traditional Mediterranean meals and learn how they alone can make wonderful lunches and dinners.

Master main-course recipes and learn the role that each dish plays in authentic Mediterranean meals.

Discover the pivotal role that fruits, cheeses, nuts, and desserts play in the Mediterranean lifestyle.

Chapter 16

What to Serve and When to Serve It

This chapter gets to the core of what the healthful Mediterranean cultures have traditionally eaten and when. Because the Mediterranean region is so large and the foods served there are so diverse, it helps to know how and when things are eaten. In this chapter, I fill you in on what makes a typical Mediterranean meal and give you some menus to try from throughout the region. I also offer tips on getting the most out of your leftovers.

Diving into Authentic Mediterranean Meals

The great thing about Mediterranean main dishes — other than their flavor and nutritional benefits — is that they can be eaten at lunch or dinner. In other words, there really aren't specific types of main dishes associated with dinner or others with lunch. In pretty much all of the various cultures in the region, Mediterranean mains are fair game to serve at either meal.

What does differ, however, is the quantity served at the main meal of the day (which is lunch) and the quantity served at dinner. For example, in Italy, lunch might begin with appetizers, followed by an essential first course (usually pasta, gnocchi, risotto, or soup), a main dish, a side dish, and then a salad. On the other hand, at dinner (on a typical weeknight at home), just the main dish and maybe a salad would be served. In many Mediterranean countries, dinners can consist of lighter items, such as soups and salads, smaller portions of main dishes, and sometimes even simple "dry" items like bread, cheese, and cured meats. Alternately, the same items that were served at lunch, but in smaller portions, may be served.

The two exceptions to the lighter-dinner rule:

>> **Entertaining:** There is such a high premium placed on entertaining in the Mediterranean that it supersedes all other customs of what to serve and when. In Arabic, there is a saying that "the food equals the affection." In most places throughout the Mediterranean basin, regardless of what language is spoken, that's the attitude. Traditionally, people have gone to great lengths to treat their guests to the best food they have available and as much of it as possible. The goal is to shower your guest with edible affection and satisfy any culinary needs they may have so they never have to ask for anything, go away hungry, or leave feeling as if they weren't taken care of. In most places throughout the region, it's considered poor manners to ask for things — even a glass of water — in someone's home, so it truly is up to the host to ensure that all of their guests' needs are met.

>> **Eating out:** Eating out in the Mediterranean region was traditionally not a regular part of daily life, the way it is in the United States. As a result, when people *do* eat out, they normally tend not to cut corners when it comes to calories. Instead, they splurge and sample the best items on the menu, just for the experience. Then, when they're at home the next night, they might have a bowl of homemade lentil soup for dinner, instead of a main course. I have some Italian friends who only eat fruit or a salad at night after enjoying a large restaurant lunch.

Exploring Mediterranean Menus

Let seasonality and your own personal tastes and schedule determine how to create menus. If you need some inspiration, here are a few menu suggestions using recipes from this book:

» Southern Italian Sunday supper:

- Antipasto platter

- Pasta al Forno con Melanzane e Caciocavallo (Baked Pasta with Eggplant and Caciocavallo; see Chapter 19)

- Agnello al Forno in Pignata (Southern Italian Lamb Stew; see Chapter 19)

- Fresh bread

- Cannellini Beans with Artichoke Hearts and Dandelion Greens (see Chapter 18)

- Apple, Almond, and Olive Oil Cake (see Chapter 20)

» Moroccan feast:

- Rustic Moroccan Barley Bread (see Chapter 17) and preserved lemons

- Moroccan Vegetable Salad Sampler (see Chapter 18)

- Tajine Djaj bil Couscous (Moroccan Chicken, Almond, and Olive Tajine with Couscous; see Chapter 19)

- Rose Water–Infused Fruit Salad (see Chapter 20)

» Spanish fiesta:

- Bread, almonds, olives, and extra-virgin olive oil

- Pollo alla Amontillado con Patatas Arrugadas y Pico Mahon (Spanish Sherry Chicken with Potatoes in Mojo Picón Sauce; see Chapter 19)

- Broccoli Rabe with Garlic, Extra-Virgin Olive Oil, and Chilies (see Chapter 18)

- Spanish Fruit, Nut, and Cheese Plate (see Chapter 20)

» Levantine taverna-style lunch:

- Tahini Sauce, Hummus, and Baba Ghanouj Trio (see Chapter 18)

- Yachni (Greek Tomato and Vegetable Stew; see Chapter 19) with Rustic Moroccan Barley Bread (see Chapter 17)

- Watermelon with Feta and Mint (see Chapter 20)

» Italian seaside dinner:

- Assorted Sicilian olives

- Pesce alla Siciliana con Verdure al Forno (Roasted Sicilian-Style Fish with Vegetables; see Chapter 19)

- Cannellini Beans with Artichoke Hearts and Dandelion Greens (see Chapter 18)

- Calabrian-Style Figs with Ricotta and Honey (see Chapter 20)

» Elegant weeknight vegetarian dinner

- Purslane with Beans, Lemon, Garlic, and Mint (see Chapter 18)

- Frittata di Carciofi, Asparagi, e Cipolle Caramellate (Artichoke, Asparagus, and Caramelized Onion Frittata; see Chapter 19)

- Provençal Cheese Platter (see Chapter 20)

» Mediterranean island dinner:

- Shrimp with Lentils and Garlic (see Chapter 18)

- Cassola de Pisci a S'Ozzastrina (Sardinian Fish Stew; see Chapter 19) with toasted bread

- Date, Walnut, and Orange Torta (see Chapter 20)

Repurposing Leftovers

You can tell a lot from a cook by the way they treat leftovers. My close friends and clients tease me that my leftovers are better than my original meals, and that's music to my ears! In the Mediterranean region, any cook — whether they're a professional or a home cook — knows numerous ways to repurpose leftovers into highly anticipated dishes.

This tradition stems from the fact that waste wasn't an option in antiquity. Even if people have the luxury of not using up every bit of an animal or a vegetable, it's still considered a waste and disrespectful to throw so much away. To this day, if I drop a piece of bread or have to throw dough out for some reason, I pick it up and hold it to my lips and then my forehead, out of respect, before tossing it into the trash. Some of my Mediterranean chef colleagues do this as well.

Until very recently, in the United States, being resourceful with food was seen as a sign that you were poor or, worse yet, cheap. Fortunately, however, many well-known restaurant chefs, celebrities, and movements have been created to promote a "zero food waste" policy, which is completely in line with the Mediterranean culture. The negative stigma about being resourceful is transforming into a powerful and socially responsible ethos.

TIP

Here's a list of dishes that I turn to time and time again to repurpose leftovers and add variety to small plates:

» **Monday salad:** *Insalata del Lunedì* is a traditional Italian housewife's way of making good use of leftovers from Sunday. The Monday salad, as it's called, is similar to a chef's salad, incorporating piles of greens with the leftover bits of meat and vegetables from Sunday, in addition to croutons made from the day-old bread.

» **Minestra:** An Italian *minestra* is a soup that contains a grain (such as pasta, rice, barley, or farro) along with chopped vegetables, stock, and various legumes. In Calabria, Italy, we make a version called *Millecosedde,* which in dialect means "a thousand little things" because it's made on New Year's Eve as a way to clear out the cupboards and the fridge for the new year. Most soups are a great way to use leftovers. Start by sautéing diced celery, diced carrot, and diced onion in extra-virgin olive oil; then add grains, vegetables, and legumes, and cover with one of the homemade stocks in Chapter 19. Slowly simmer the soup until the grains and legumes are tender.

» **Skillet shwarma:** *Shwarma* is popular rotisserie meat that's stuffed into pitas or served thinly sliced over rice in the Middle East. You can make a mouthwatering version at home with leftover bits of meat or chicken. Just use the shredded protein of your choice. In a large skillet, sauté an onion and a green bell pepper in a bit of olive oil. When the vegetables are soft, add the meat and your favorite seasonings. I also add a few chopped-up tomatoes (just enough to make the mixture wet) and sauté it for a few minutes. Stuff the mixture into pita pockets and dress with tahini sauce.

» **Frittatas or omelets:** In the Southern European portion of the Mediterranean (such as France, Italy, and Spain), omelets, tortillas, and frittatas are eaten for lunch or dinner, not at breakfast. If you have leftover meat, beans, or vegetables, you can add them to these three classics. You can use the Frittata di Carciofi, Asparagi, e Cipolle Caramellate (Artichoke, Asparagus, and Caramelized Onion Frittata) recipe in Chapter 19 as a guide, adding in your own leftovers instead of the artichokes and asparagus.

» **Ravioli:** In Italy, crafty cooks have been chopping or pureeing leftovers into homemade ravioli filling for hundreds of years. The bonus to this idea is that you get to sample additional varieties instead of just the regular spinach, meat, and cheese.

» **Savory pies and pizza:** Every Mediterranean country has its own tradition of savory pies, from Greece's Spanakopita (Savory Greek Spinach Pie; Chapter 17) to Turkey's *pide* (hand-stretched flatbreads with savory toppings) and Italy's *pizza rustica* (savory pies filled with greens, cheese, and/or meat). You can also use leftovers to top pizza or make stuffed pizza dough (calzones). So, whether you prefer phyllo dough, quiche dough, or pizza dough, wrapping your leftovers in a new way is an edible present for the taste buds.

>> **Sformato:** A *sformato* is a molded Italian appetizer, akin to a savory flan, that's easy to make and impressive to serve. To make *sformato,* puree leftover vegetables in a food processor. Add plain breadcrumbs and cheese, if needed, and herbs of your choice, to form a thick, pastelike consistency. Grease individual ramekins and fill three-fourths full with the *sformato* paste. Bake at 350 degrees until set, about 15 minutes, and turn out on a plate. Depending on the vegetable you're using, you could spoon an appropriate sauce — such as tomato, pesto, or cheese — over top.

>> **Gratin:** Gratin-style vegetables aren't as popular in the United States nowadays as they were when I was growing up, but I hope they make a comeback! France is still known for them, and many Mediterranean countries make good use of them, too. Gratin is a culinary technique in which your vegetable of choice is topped with breadcrumbs, grated cheese, eggs, and butter and baked in a shallow dish until golden on top. You can make one out of a main vegetable and then incorporate leftover bits in the dish.

>> **Purees, dips, and *veloutés*:** I always use leftover beans, vegetables, and lentils this way. If I want to make a simple dip, I just put them in a food processor and add some extra-virgin olive oil, citrus juice, herbs, and spices to taste, thinning it out with a little water if needed, until I have a delicious dip or puree that I can serve with crudités or pita chips. To make a *velouté* soup, I add homemade stock (see Chapter 19) until I have the desired thickness and let it simmer on the stove for a few minutes before serving it with bread or homemade croutons.

Chapter **17**

Breakfast

Most of what you find floating around the Internet in terms of "Mediterranean recipes" are actually American-style dishes with Mediterranean ingredients. This approach is fine, and some of the dishes can be quite tasty. but in order to really embrace and enjoy the Mediterranean lifestyle, authentic dishes from the region can provide endless inspiration.

In this chapter, I explain what breakfast looks like in various Mediterranean countries, give you ideas for quick breakfasts, and offer recipes for when you have a bit more time to linger over breakfast.

Starting Your Day the Sunny Mediterranean Way

You can learn a lot about a culture and their meal patterns from the way they start their day. Even though the different countries in the Mediterranean enjoy different breakfast foods and styles, there is one thing that binds them together: starting the day with flavorful inspiration.

If you've been to a Mediterranean country and stayed in a hotel, the breakfast you sampled there was probably a combination of a few local favorites with a wide variety of American and continental favorites, and not a true representation of the local traditions.

In the Mediterranean, the biggest meal happens at midday, so breakfast is really just a bridge, giving you enough nutrients to start your day with a boost of energy, but not weighing you down.

What breakfast looks like throughout the Mediterranean

Breakfast varies from one country to the next, throughout the Mediterranean. The following sections walk you through how breakfast differs in a variety of Mediterranean countries.

Egypt

Traditional breakfasts in Egypt are very large and varied. The most emblematic food of the nation is *fuul medammes* (stewed fava beans), which is also a popular snack and street food. Sometimes *fuul medammes* is served as lunch or dinner by those with less money, as well as by vegetarians and vegans everywhere who appreciate global cuisine. Packed with protein and spiced with flavor, they're eaten everywhere with *aish baladi* (the local hot, fresh, pita bread dusted with crushed bran). Egyptians also use fava beans to make *t'ameya* (the fava bean falafel recipe eaten by the Coptic Christian community since ancient times during Lent). Eggs, fresh vegetables (cucumber, tomato, carrot, and green onion), pickled vegetables, cheeses, and tahini sauce are also common at the Egyptian breakfast table.

The Egyptians accompany this meal with black tea (usually with mint) and sometimes follow it with Turkish coffee. A sweetened wheat or rice pudding can often be served in place of what Americans eat for cereal. But the dishes I mention here are often just the beginning. Sometimes an assortment of breads, butter, and jams; a flaky homemade pastry called *fateer m'sheltit*; sweetened clotted cream; honey; and fruits can also be included. On weekends and holidays, Egyptians may even follow their breakfast with dessert.

Egyptians typically eat lunch much later in the day, and this large breakfast helps to keep them satisfied until then.

Greece

Breakfasts in the Hellenic Republic bridge the culinary gap between East and West. In Greece, you can enjoy freshly baked croissants and sweet cream-filled pastries such as *bougatsa* or opt for the savory spinach- or cheese-stuffed pita pastries accompanied with fresh fruit and juices. Greek coffee and, nowadays, espresso and American coffee are also becoming popular. Some prefer a simple start to their day with Greek yogurt slathered with natural Greek honey. Freshly baked bread, often studded with sesame seeds, is another typical option.

Israel

I've heard it said that if you eat an Israeli breakfast, you won't need lunch. Israelis start their day in a manner as varied as the country's ethnic makeup itself. In Israel, you can also enjoy a wide range of both sweet and savory dishes. Shakshouka, brought to Israel by Tunisian Jews, is the best known; it features eggs simmered in peppers and tomato sauce. Traditional Arab foods, such as chopped salads, hummus, tahini sauce, cheese, fava bean puree, baba ghanouj, yogurt with honey, and strained yogurt (known as labneh) are all popular. Fresh, hot pita bread, eggs, and cold and hot cereals made with semolina and oatmeal are also enjoyed.

Ashkenazi influences of smoked fish, soft cheeses, and blintzes are also common choices. Add in vegetable soufflés, pancakes, and waffles along with other continental classics, and you truly have a world of choices to start your day with. Coffee, tea, and fresh juices accompany breakfast, and Israelis can also choose to complete the first meal of the day with dessert (if they saved room!).

Italy

Italian breakfasts are short and sweet. Literally. Breakfast in Italy causes a lot of confusion for Americans, who see it as carb-heavy and nutritionally incomplete. But Italians don't think of breakfast as a way to get through the day. To an Italian, breakfast is a sweet way to charge your morning with caffeine and carbs while allowing you to enjoy a complete, delicious, and varied lunch at midday. *Cornetti* (Italian croissants made with a sourdough starter), toast rusks, biscotti (not the twice-baked variety you may be thinking of, but breakfast cookies), fruit, juices, and, of course, coffee — in the form of espresso, a caffe latte, or a cappuccino — are what the majority of Italians start their day with.

Many American cookbooks on Mediterranean food describe frittatas as an Italian breakfast, but Italians don't find the idea of eating eggs in the morning appealing — a frittata, in Italy, is served at dinner. In addition to being much lighter than the North African and Middle Eastern breakfasts, an Italian breakfast is usually not lingered over. Even on weekends, breakfast is still light, and the extra time is all focused on lunch, especially on Sundays. In Italian bars (cafés that also serve alcohol), people eat their coffee and pastry standing up, in a matter of minutes, before jetting off to work, school, or play.

The Levant: Cyprus, Lebanon, Jordan, Palestine, and Turkey

The eastern portion of the Mediterranean is known for ample breakfasts, with sweet and savory dishes. Many of the dishes that I mention in the "Egypt" and "Israel" sections are also popular in the Levant, but breakfast tables in the Levant have some additional favorites.

In Cyprus, for example, olives, fried or grilled halloumi or Anari cheese, along with *lountza* (Cypriot bacon or sausage), are served with sesame-seed-covered bread, along with local yogurt and honey.

In Lebanon, it's labneh, the creamy, tangy, yogurt cheese drizzled with local olive oil and served with herbs, vegetables, and fresh hot pita bread that stands out. Palestinians make a za'atar-covered flatbread called *mannqish,* which is a delicious snack to eat anytime but is often enjoyed hot out of the oven, slathered with labneh, and topped with an egg.

For Turks, the word for breakfast, *kahvalti,* comes from the root word, *kahva,* which means coffee. The feast happens daily — weekend or not. Cheeses, *simit* (sesame studded hard bread rings that look like bagels). Homemade jams and honey, eggs, beef sausage, vegetables, and olives are usually present. Despite the coffee connection in the name for breakfast, many Turks drink black tea after starting their day instead of coffee.

Morocco

The staple items from other North African and Middle Eastern countries — such as eggs, cheese, vegetables, bread, preserves, and honey — are also part of Moroccan breakfasts. Some unique griddle breads called *m'semen* (homemade puff pastry made with aged clarified butter), *harcha* (round cornmeal cakes), *beghrir* (honeycomb pancakes that are perfect for soaking up honey), and homemade doughnuts called *sfenj* (sponges) are the highlights in my mind. For dessert, rice- and couscous-based puddings, as well as rice-pudding-stuffed pastry triangles that are fried and topped with cinnamon, and traditional Moroccan cookies are present.

Spain

The Spanish *desayuno* (breakfast) can often be a lighter fare like the Italian breakfast, but it offers savory variations as well. At home, Spaniards usually eat *galletas* (biscuits) or muffin-type pastries known as *magdalenas* with a cup of *café* (coffee) or *café con leche* (coffee with milk). Outside, you can choose from *churros con chocolate* (fried-choux pastry sticks or rings) served with a cup of thick, hot chocolate for dipping, *tostadas* (toasted bread with different toppings), *tortilla Española* (potato omelet), or *bocadillos* (sandwiches served on French bread that are usually filled with Spanish ham or cheeses).

What makes a "good" breakfast

If you read the previous sections, you may be salivating and wondering how all these delicious foods could be part of a healthful lifestyle! I actually rejoiced when I learned the nutritional advantages of adopting these eating styles.

Remember the Ancient Greek philosopher Cleobulus's saying: "Moderation is best."

Choose the breakfast style that fits in with your tastes, lifestyle, and eating patterns. If you're going to skip lunch, for example, the heavier Israeli, Egyptian, or Levantine breakfasts may serve you well. If your lunches happen early and provide a lot of nutritional and caloric content, the Italian breakfast or simple, dairy fresh yogurt with honey and fruit will be all you need.

Research has shown that eating a large breakfast in the morning can reduce your appetite throughout the day and help you lose weight. One study showed that overweight women with *metabolic syndrome* (a cluster of conditions including high blood pressure, high blood sugar, high cholesterol, and too much body fat around the waist) were able to lose weight and belly fat better by eating a big breakfast than by following a conventional 1,400-calorie diet. The larger breakfast was also shown to prevent diabetes and heart disease. Additional research has shown that those who eat a big breakfast burn twice as many calories as those who eat a larger dinner. Eating a big breakfast has also been linked to improved mood and metabolism, as well as better food choices throughout the day. Starting the day with 30 grams of protein is actually recommended by neuro-therapists for optimal brain function.

It's up to you to decide (perhaps with the help of a dietitian or nutritionist) which breakfast plan works for you. I like to switch it up, depending on my schedule. When I work from home, I follow the "lunch as the largest meal of the day" Mediterranean tradition, so I can get by with a smaller breakfast. Often when I'm traveling or cooking for a TV show or a large-scale event and I know I might not get lunch, I have a larger breakfast. Weekdays and days off are fun times to experiment with more elaborate recipes.

Grabbing Breakfast on the Go

Maybe the thought of making breakfast while you're trying to get the kids off to school is too much. Maybe you've got a long commute and have to be out the door bright and early. Maybe you're just not a "breakfast person" or you'd rather spend the time exercising or meditating in the morning. Whatever your reason for not wanting a long, drawn-out breakfast, the following list is for you.

TIP

Here are some grab-and-go breakfasts to have on hand:

>> A serving of Greek yogurt with fruit or crudités

>> A handful of almonds and an orange

>> A serving of labneh and a piece of whole-wheat pita bread with dates

>> A hard-boiled egg, a handful of walnuts, and a piece of aged cheese

>> A serving of whole-milk ricotta with a drizzle of local honey

>> A serving of overnight oats with fresh fruit

>> A serving of fresh fruit salad with a few tablespoons of Greek yogurt

>> A smoothie made out of ½ cup Greek yogurt, 1 ripe banana, ½ cup strawberry slices, and a few ice cubes

Instead of turning to fast food or sugary cereals on a busy morning, or skipping breakfast even though you're really hungry, keep these formulas and foods on hand to carry you to lunchtime. Enjoy them with a sense of gratitude, and look forward to whatever part of your day brings you the most joy!

Enjoying a Leisurely Breakfast

In addition to making great rituals and recipes, the dishes in this section, with the exception of the Pan di Spagna (Italian Sponge Cake), make great, quick, vegetarian dinners. Instead of going through the drive-thru or ordering out, if you come home hungry and short on time, turn to these options for supper. Serve the sponge cake with berries for dessert!

Homemade Labneh Cheese

PREP TIME: ABOUT 1 MIN PLUS 12–24 HR FOR RESTING	COOK TIME: NONE	YIELD: 4 SERVINGS

INGREDIENTS

4 cups plain, full-fat Greek yogurt

1 teaspoon unrefined sea salt

¼ cup Amy Riolo Selections Extra-Virgin Olive Oil or other good-quality extra-virgin olive oil

Fresh mint, for garnish (optional)

DIRECTIONS

1 In a cheese cloth or a fine-mesh strainer that sits easily in another bowl, place the yogurt.

2 Mix in the salt and strain for 12 hours. (If you prefer your labneh thick, strain it for 24 hours.)

3 Transfer the labneh from the strainer to a storage container with a tight-fitting lid. Reserve the liquid to drink later (see the following Tip).

4 To serve, spoon the labneh onto 4 plates and flatten with the back of a spoon. Use the spoon to make indentations, and drizzle 1 tablespoon olive oil over each serving.

5 Garnish with fresh mint, if desired.

PER SERVING: *Calories 333 (From Fat 218); Fat 24g (Saturated 9g); Cholesterol 0mg; Sodium 662mg; Carbohydrate 11g (Dietary Fiber 0g); Protein 20g.*

TIP: The reserved liquid from straining the water is highly praised in Mediterranean households and often served as a tonic to those who need a healthy dose of probiotics and inulin, which is believed to balance blood sugar levels.

NOTE: Labneh, bread, and dates are among the world's oldest foods. For centuries, nomads made yogurt and yogurt cheese by beating milk in between animal hides hung on trees. They supplemented their daily diet with bread and dates. Because yogurt contains all three macronutrients (carbohydrate, protein, and fat), it makes a nutritious breakfast or snack all by itself. The name of the country Lebanon comes from the plural form of the word *labneh* in Arabic (which is *lebnan*). Many Middle Eastern markets sell packaged varieties, but making your own is fun and inexpensive, and the result is fresher!

VARY IT! Warm pita bread topped with labneh and eggs is a common breakfast in the Levant region of the Mediterranean. To make it, you can heat a whole piece of pita bread, smear it with labneh, and top with chopped hardboiled eggs or poached eggs. Or you can sprinkle pita with za'atar and crack an egg on top and bake it. My favorite way to eat labneh is drizzled with olive oil served with pita chips, tomato chunks, cucumber slices, and fresh mint.

Spanakopita (Savory Greek Spinach Pie)

PREP TIME: 30 MIN PLUS 30 MIN FOR RESTING	COOK TIME: 45 MIN	YIELD: 4 SERVINGS

INGREDIENTS

15 ounces fresh spinach, washed, dried, and finely chopped

½ cup washed and chopped leek bulbs (white part only) or diced onion

1 cup crumbled feta cheese

2 tablespoons ricotta cheese

Freshly ground black pepper to taste

1 bunch fresh mint, finely chopped

1 bunch fresh dill, finely chopped

Zest of 1 lemon

3 eggs, whisked in a small bowl until frothy

2 cups unbleached all-purpose flour, plus extra for kneading

½ cup plus 1 teaspoon Amy Riolo Selections Extra-Virgin Olive Oil or other good-quality extra-virgin olive oil, divided

1 tablespoon white wine vinegar

1 teaspoon unrefined sea salt

¾ cup lukewarm water

2 tablespoons cornstarch

¼ cup unsalted butter

DIRECTIONS

1   Preheat the oven to 400 degrees.

2   Make the filling by combining the spinach, leek or onion, feta, ricotta, black pepper, mint, dill, and lemon zest. Stir in the eggs until well incorporated. Set aside.

3   To make the dough, in a large bowl, add the flour, 1 tablespoon of the olive oil, the vinegar, and the sea salt, and stir. Add the lukewarm water, and continue stirring, until the dough forms a ball. Add a bit more lukewarm water, 1 tablespoon at a time if needed.

4   Scatter a bit of flour onto a clean work surface and knead the dough until smooth, about 5 to 10 minutes. Wrap the dough in plastic wrap and allow to rest at room temperature for 30 minutes to 3 hours.

5   When you're ready to continue, dust a clean work surface with a bit of flour. Unwrap the dough, and roll it into an even log shape, approximately 10 inches long. Cut the log into 8 equally sized pieces. Roll each piece into a ball. Place on a plate or baking sheet, and cover with plastic wrap to prevent the dough balls from drying out.

6   Dust the work surface again. Coat the first dough ball lightly with cornstarch and a bit of flour. Flatten out the dough ball with your hands into a disk. Roll out the dough ball with a rolling pin into a flat circle, about 5 inches in diameter. Repeat with the rest of the dough, trying to make them as close to the same size as possible.

7   Grease a 10-inch pie pan with 1 teaspoon of olive oil. Set aside.

8   In a saucepan, melt the butter. Stir in the remaining 3 tablespoons of olive oil.

9 Place 1 dough circle onto a plate, and brush to cover with the olive oil and butter mixture. Repeat with 4 more circles, brushing each in between, and placing them in a stack. Do not brush the top layer with oil. Press down on the edges of the stack, sealing with your fingers. Place the plate in the refrigerator to chill while you repeat the same process with the remaining 3 dough balls on a separate plate. Chill those as well.

10 Take the 5 layers of stacked dough out of the fridge and place on a lightly floured work surface. With a rolling pin, roll out each layer to a 12-inch diameter.

11 To pick up the dough circle, roll it lightly around a dusted rolling pin and lay it into the pan with the excess over the edge. Drizzle with olive oil. Repeat the same process with the 3 layers on the separate plate.

12 Spoon the filling onto the dough that's already lining the pan, and smooth out the top.

13 Place the remaining dough on the top and crimp the borders of dough together to form a crust. Brush the tops with melted butter and/or oil and make evenly sized squares or diamonds by cutting pie three-fourths of the way down.

14 Bake for about 45 minutes or until the top layer of dough is golden and crisp.

15 Cool to almost room temperature and serve.

PER SERVING: *Calories 802 (From Fat 479); Fat 53g (Saturated 19g); Cholesterol 226mg; Sodium 1,157mg; Carbohydrate 62g (Dietary Fiber 6g); Protein 21g.*

NOTE: This recipe (minus the feta cheese) is traditional during Orthodox Lent, when believers follow a vegan diet. That version usually includes bulgur wheat and additional vegetables instead of the cheese and eggs. The dough can be topped with olive oil instead of butter.

NOTE: Hortopita (greens pie), spanakopita (spinach pie), and tiropita (cheese pie) are the most common savory pies (known as pita) in Greece. In addition to being eaten for breakfast and as a snack, these scrumptious treats can also be part of lunch or dinner or served as an appetizer.

VARY IT! If you want to swap out the spinach for another green, such as Swiss chard or dandelion greens, this recipe will still work well. You can also create your own fillings with leftover chicken, meat, and/or beans.

Pan di Spagna (Italian Sponge Cake)

| PREP TIME: ABOUT 15 MIN | COOK TIME: 40 MIN | YIELD: 8 SERVINGS |

INGREDIENTS

6 large egg whites

1 cup sugar

6 large egg yolks

2 teaspoons vanilla

1 cup plus 2 tablespoons unbleached all-purpose flour

1 cup apricot preserves

Powdered sugar, for dusting

DIRECTIONS

1 Preheat the oven to 350 degrees. Grease a 1½-quart loaf pan (8¼ x 9 x 2¾ inch) with olive oil spray.

2 In a large bowl, beat the egg whites until stiff peaks form. Set aside.

3 In a bowl, add the sugar and egg yolks and beat until the mixture is very light yellow in color. Stir in the vanilla. Gently fold the egg whites into the batter. Sprinkle the flour on top of the mixture and carefully incorporate the flour into the batter until just combined.

4 Pour the batter into the prepared baking pan and bake until the cake is golden and the sides begin to pull away from the pan, about 40 minutes. Remove from the oven and allow to cool completely.

5 To serve, slice in half horizontally and slather the middle of the cake with the apricot preserves. Top and sprinkle with powdered sugar. Serve in 1-inch-thick wedges.

PER SERVING: *Calories 326 (From Fat 36); Fat 4g (Saturated 1g); Cholesterol 159mg; Sodium 69mg; Carbohydrate 68g (Dietary Fiber 1g); Protein 7g.*

NOTE: This is a classic Italian cake eaten for breakfast, as a snack, or as a base for more elaborate holiday desserts. It's also a delicious base for shortcakes and sundaes. You can double the recipe and freeze one cake wrapped in plastic wrap for another time.

NOTE: This soft, quintessential Italian cake is called Pan di Spagna (literally, Bread of Spain) because it was first created in the 17th century in Madrid by a Ligurian cook, Giovan Battista Cabona (also known as Giobatta). The cook to the Spanish courts was inspired by Portuguese biscuits and lady-fingers and came up with the "new" dessert, which the Spanish royal courts baptized as a Genoise cake (or cake from Genova, the capital of Giobatta's region). To this day, the rest of the world calls the cake Genoise, while Italians refer to it as Pan di Spagna. In addition to homemade versions, most pastry shops sell it in a wide range of varieties, and supermarkets sell packaged versions in single servings in the breakfast aisles. Instead of a row of cereal, like American stores have, Italian markets have countless varieties of breakfast cookies, biscuits, and pan di Spagna.

VARY IT! For a chocolate sponge, add ½ cup fair trade cocoa powder to the batter with the sugar.

Rustic Moroccan Barley Bread

<table>
<tr><td>PREP TIME: ABOUT 20 MIN PLUS 1 HR FOR RISING</td><td>COOK TIME: 30 MIN</td><td>YIELD: 18 SERVINGS</td></tr>
</table>

INGREDIENTS

2½ cups warm water

1 tablespoon active, dry yeast

2 teaspoons honey

1 teaspoon kosher salt

6 to 8 cups barley flour, plus extra for kneading

4 teaspoons Amy Riolo Selections Extra-Virgin Olive Oil or other good-quality extra-virgin olive oil, divided

3 teaspoons sesame seeds

DIRECTIONS

1 In a large bowl, add the warm water. Sprinkle the yeast over the water, and mix until dissolved. Add the honey and salt.

2 Gradually mix in 6 cups of flour, with a wooden spoon, adding up to 2 more cups, 1 cup at a time, if needed, until the dough pulls away from the side of the bowl.

3 When the dough becomes a ball, turn it out onto a flour-dusted surface and knead until smooth, about 5 to 10 minutes. Roll the dough into a 12-inch log; then divide into three equal pieces.

4 Shape each piece into a 4-inch dome-shaped loaf. Grease a baking sheet with 1 teaspoon of the oil. Place the loaves on the baking sheet. Cover with a kitchen towel and place in a draft-free area to rise until doubled, about 1 hour.

5 Preheat the oven to 350 degrees. Uncover the loaves and brush each loaf with 1 teaspoon olive oil, and sprinkle with 1 teaspoon sesame seeds.

6 Bake until lightly golden, about 20 to 30 minutes. Let cool slightly, and serve warm.

PER SERVING: *Calories 186 (From Fat 19); Fat 2g (Saturated 0g); Cholesterol 0mg; Sodium 132mg; Carbohydrate 38g (Dietary Fiber 5g); Protein 6g.*

NOTE: The ingredients list calls for 6 to 8 cups of flour because the amount that you need will depend on how finely milled the flour is, as well as the temperature and humidity level of the room that you're baking in. When I make this recipe in Morocco, it's usually much drier, so I need less flour (closer to 6 cups). In Washington, D.C., however, where I live, we have notoriously humid summers, and I've used up to 8 cups of flour when baking it. Let your fingers be your guide, and start out with 6 cups of flour, only adding a bit more at a time until the dough no longer sticks to the surface while kneading.

TIP: This bread is great for any meal, Moroccan or not. It would make a good accompaniment to most main dishes and small plates in this book.

NOTE: This bread is best eaten the day it's made, or frozen and then defrosted and reheated the day it's served. Freeze by wrapping it in plastic wrap and then aluminum foil. Thaw at room temperature and warm in a preheated 350-degree oven before serving.

VARY IT! You don't have to use barley flour in this recipe. White flour, whole-wheat flour, or ½ of each work really well. In Morocco, many families make this bread with a natural sourdough starter (also made from barley). If you happen to make your own starter, you can use it in this recipe.

Egyptian Fuul Medammes with Tahini

PREP TIME: ABOUT 2 MIN	COOK TIME: 5 MIN	YIELD: 4 SERVINGS

INGREDIENTS

2 teaspoons Amy Riolo Selections Extra-Virgin Olive Oil or other good-quality extra-virgin olive oil, divided

One 15-ounce can cooked fava beans with juice

½ teaspoon cumin

½ teaspoon dried ground coriander

⅛ teaspoon salt

Freshly ground black pepper to taste

¼ cup tahini sauce

4 pieces pita bread, for serving

DIRECTIONS

1 In a medium frying map, add 1 teaspoon of the olive oil and warm over medium–low heat. Add the beans and juice from the can, the cumin, the coriander, the salt, and the pepper. Stir well to combine. Cook until most of the liquid has absorbed, about 5 minutes.

2 Reduce the heat to low and mash slightly with a fork or potato masher, cooking just until the mixture is slightly looser than refried beans, about 1 minute. Serve immediately.

3 Spoon onto a serving plate. Drizzle with tahini sauce. Make a hole in the center and drizzle the remaining 1 teaspoon of olive oil into it. Serve with pita bread.

PER SERVING: *Calories 204 (From Fat 96); Fat 11g (Saturated 1g); Cholesterol 0mg; Sodium 612mg; Carbohydrate 20g (Dietary Fiber 5g); Protein 9g.*

TIP: Cooked fava beans, or *fuul medammes,* can be found online or in Middle Eastern markets.

TIP: Tahini sauce (you can find a recipe in Chapter 18) is a classic way to top *fuul,* but the beans themselves are a blank culinary canvas for lots of toppings — just like baked potatoes or nachos are in the United States. Restaurants and food carts selling *fuul* will give you your choice of diced fresh vegetables (tomato, cucumber, onion), olive oil and lemon, crumbled egg, and other options for enjoying them in addition to this version.

NOTE: Protein- and fiber-dense fava beans are believed to be the world's oldest agricultural crop — they're said to have been one of the pharaoh's favorites. This traditional Egyptian dish is still a popular breakfast and snack food. Recently, Egyptian doctors released research proving that a breakfast of fava bean puree, eggs, and pita bread provides all the nutrients needed during a day's worth of activity.

NOTE: Most people in the region prefer dried beans to canned, but *fuul* are an exception. Large, skin-on, dried fava beans take *hours* to cook. In Egypt, they use a *demassa* (a long cylindrical vessel with a narrow opening) for slow-cooking the beans up to 8 hours. If you have a slow cooker and can find the dried beans, you can do it this way. Of all the Egyptians I met, only one made them at home from the dried version. The rest used the canned variety or purchased them precooked.

Bileela (Creamy Wheatberry Cereal)

PREP TIME: ABOUT 5 MIN PLUS OVERNIGHT FOR SOAKING	COOK TIME: NONE	YIELD: 4 SERVINGS

INGREDIENTS

1 cup whole white wheatberries (pearl, soft, or hard), rinsed

⅓ cup sugar or honey, or to taste

½ cup warm milk

½ cup raisins or other dried fruit (optional)

DIRECTIONS

1 At night, place whole wheatberries in a large thermos and cover with boiling water. The next morning, the wheat will be puffed and tender.

2 Stir sugar or honey into the wheat, if desired, and spoon into 4 cereal bowls. Top with warm milk and raisins or dried fruit, if using.

PER SERVING: *Calories 270 (From Fat 14); Fat 2g (Saturated 0g); Cholesterol 2mg; Sodium 15mg; Carbohydrate 62g (Dietary Fiber 9g); Protein 8g.*

TIP: If you use hard wheat, the wheat itself will require an hour of soaking in cold water prior to preparing the recipe.

NOTE: This could very well be the world's oldest cereal recipe. Bileela is a comforting whole-wheat cereal that is enjoyed all over the Arab world. It's even sold in street-side stalls at breakfast time in plastic bags for people who don't have time to boil it at home.

VARY IT! If you want to use different types of grains, such as barley, quinoa, or rice, for a warm cereal in the morning, just prepare them according to package directions in advance. The next morning, stir in honey, dried fruits, and nuts, and enjoy.

Halloumi Mashwi bil Baid (Halloumi Cheese with Eggs, Tomatoes, Herbs, and Cucumbers)

PREP TIME: ABOUT 15 MIN	COOK TIME: 10 MIN	YIELD: 4 SERVINGS

INGREDIENTS

¼ cup Amy Riolo Selections Extra-Virgin Olive Oil or other good-quality extra-virgin olive oil

One 8-ounce package Halloumi cheese, sliced ¼-inch thick

4 large eggs

2 plum tomatoes, halved

1 teaspoon za'atar

Salt to taste

Freshly ground black pepper to taste

4 Persian cucumbers, quartered

1 bunch radishes (optional)

1 bunch fresh parsley

1 bunch fresh mint

1 bunch fresh cilantro (optional)

DIRECTIONS

1 In a large, deep, wide skillet, add the olive oil and warm over medium heat. Add the Halloumi cheese and allow to brown slightly, 3 to 5 minutes per side. Add the eggs around the cheese, and then add the tomatoes. Season with za'atar, salt, and pepper. Allow the eggs to cook to your desired doneness, about 5 to 10 minutes, covering with a lid, if necessary.

2 In the meantime, on one side of a platter, arrange the cucumbers, radishes, parsley, mint, and cilantro, if desired.

3 When the eggs are finished cooking, transfer them, along with the Halloumi and tomatoes, to the other side of the platter and enjoy immediately.

PER SERVING: *Calories 380 (From Fat 294); Fat 33g (Saturated 13g); Cholesterol 252mg; Sodium 676mg; Carbohydrate 5g (Dietary Fiber 1g); Protein 19g.*

NOTE: Cilantro and parsley help the body with detoxification and are readily found in Arab cuisine. Feel free to use your favorite herbs or green onions instead.

TIP: Serve fresh, hot bread with this dish, which tastes great and is a satisfying option any time of the day.

VARY IT! You could make the same dish and substitute hardboiled eggs for the eggs cooked with the Halloumi cheese. For a vegan alternative, use portobello mushrooms in place of the Halloumi and edamame instead of the eggs.

Green Shakshouka

PREP TIME: ABOUT 15 MIN	COOK TIME: 25 MIN	YIELD: 6 SERVINGS

INGREDIENTS

2 tablespoons Amy Riolo Selections Extra-Virgin Olive Oil or other good-quality extra-virgin olive oil

2 tablespoons harissa sauce or chili paste (optional)

2 tablespoons tomato paste

1 teaspoon za'atar

1 yellow onion, diced

2 large green bell peppers, trimmed, seeded, and cut into small pieces

3 cups chopped green tomatoes or baby spinach

6 large eggs

½ cup Homemade Labneh Cheese (see recipe earlier in this chapter) or Greek yogurt

6 slices Rustic Moroccan Barley Bread (see recipe earlier in this chapter) or other pita, warmed, for serving

DIRECTIONS

1 In a large skillet, add the olive oil and warm over medium heat. Add the harissa or chili paste, tomato paste, za'atar, onion, and peppers. Stir well to combine and allow to cook until the peppers are tender, about 5 to 7 minutes.

2 Add the tomatoes or spinach, stir, and increase the heat to high. When the mixture begins to cook down, reduce the heat to low. If using tomatoes, simmer until the sauce thickens, about 10 minutes. If using spinach, cook for just a few minutes until desired doneness is reached. Taste and adjust the seasoning with more za'atar, if desired.

3 Make 6 wells in the sauce. Break 1 egg into each well. Using a fork, gently swirl the egg whites into the sauce. Simmer, uncovered, until the egg whites are set but the egg yolks are not yet hard, about 6 to 8 minutes.

4 Remove from the heat and allow to set for a few minutes before serving. Serve with labneh or yogurt and hot bread.

PER SERVING: *Calories 243 (From Fat 98); Fat 11g (Saturated 3g); Cholesterol 212mg; Sodium 250mg; Carbohydrate 25g (Dietary Fiber 3g); Protein 12g.*

NOTE: *Shakshouka* means "mixture" in Arabic, and this dish is of Tunisian, Algerian, Moroccan, and Libyan origin; nowadays it's extremely popular in Israel, too. Variations are actually served throughout the Mediterranean region. Served for breakfast, lunch, or dinner, traditionally in a cast-iron pan, this is one of the tastiest, easiest, and most economical dishes around.

VARY IT! If you want to make the classic shakshouka recipe, use red tomatoes instead of green tomatoes, and red bell pepper instead of a green bell pepper.

Chapter 18

Small Plates and Snacks

One of my friends from Cyprus used to tell me about the delights of sitting on her large balcony in the summer during late, breezy nights. She said she would invite her friends over, and it would not be uncommon for them to serve at least 40 different small plates during the course of the evening. The combination of foods and flavors, all unassumingly presented, she said, encouraged conversation and reinforced the beauty of socialization.

This chapter explores the dazzling small plates that precede many traditional Mediterranean meals and discusses how they can be transformed into delicious and nutritious meals. I also fill you in on snacking in the Mediterranean, so you'll never again have an excuse for buying something from a vending machine!

From Tapas to Mezze and Beyond

In the Mediterranean, each country and some cities have a tradition of small plates. They also have specific customs in which they're served. Not all small plates are served late at night, for example, as the Spanish tapas are. Some are served prior to meals as appetizers (especially in the North African and Levantine portions of the Mediterranean). In Italy and France, small plates can be served as appetizers or at an afternoon aperitif, well before dinner.

TIP

Here are a few times you might like to incorporate small plates into your routine:

>> You want to experience a lot of variety in one sitting.

>> You're looking for a fun, new, entertaining theme meal.

>> You're going to be eating alfresco.

>> You're hosting a brunch, happy hour, or late-night event.

Eating from many different dishes — even in small amounts — tricks the brain into thinking that you're consuming more than you actually are. Just *seeing* that many dishes helps you to fill up faster. The variety is also satisfying and triggers feelings of calm and satiation before you even pick up your fork. Finally, the more small plates of varied foods and cooking preparations you have to choose from, the more nutrients you're likely to get in one sitting.

SMALL PLATES FROM A TO Z

Mediterranean countries have their own names for small plates. Here are a few common ones:

- **Tapas:** Tapas are a Spanish tradition. They get their name from the word *cover.* Originally, the barkeeps would cover drinks with plates to keep them clean. Hungry customers requested food on the plates, and the notion of small plates being offered to accompany food took on this name. In Spain, unlike other places in the Mediterranean, tapas can become a movable feast. Instead of spending dinner in one place, people move from one tapas bar to another, sampling the best that each place has to offer throughout the night. Some of my friends and I would have tapas parties when we lived in the same neighborhood. Each of us would prepare a few different dishes, and we would all go from house to house sampling them.

- **Antipasto/aperitive:** In Italian cities other than Venice, small plates can come from the traditional *antipasti,* which are literally appetizers served prior to a meal, or *aperitive,* which are small nibbles served to accompany a cocktail or prosecco at the end of the workday (but still several hours before dinner). In Italy, if you want to extend your time with someone, you can invite them to an aperitive prior to dinner. Much lighter dishes — such as nuts, olives, and olive oil crackers (or even potato chips nowadays) — are served at the aperitive. Some places specialize in mini pizzas, risotto croquettes, and cheese and meat boards as well.

- **Hors d'oeuvres/aperitif:** In France, as in Italy, small plates come both as appetizers or *amuse-bouches* (literally, "mouth pleasers") or to accompany the afternoon aperitif. It's very common for the French to entertain by inviting friends over for an aperitif, even if they don't intend to eat dinner together.

- *Cichetti:* Venice, Italy, has its own brand of small plates called *cichetti.* Bar owners used to need to come up with quick and filling dishes to feed the gondoliers when they would come in for a drink and respite from the hot sun. Nowadays, these dishes are their own tradition. Chefs love making *cichetti* because they're a great way to repurpose food in a professional kitchen. What's even better is that, in traditional Italian cooking, there isn't much room for variance. With *cichetti,* however, chefs get to unleash their creative sides and elevate little bits of foods to new heights.

- *Salatat:* Though it literally means "salads," *salatat* is the Arabic word for the small plates of beans, legumes, cooked and raw vegetable salads, pickles, and olives set out at restaurants prior to large meals.

- *Mezze:* In Lebanon, *mezze* were first served in roadside tavernas in the Bekkah Valley where hungry travelers stopped for sustenance. Since then, they've flourished and grown to full-blown meal status, often incorporating hot and cold, vegetarian, and meat dishes all in one sitting. Because there are more Lebanese people living around the world than in the small country itself, Lebanese cuisine has become a global favorite. Its *mezze* are what Lebanon is most internationally recognized for.

  Other countries in the Levant also serve *mezze* as a means to accompany alcohol. In the cases of Greece, Cyprus, and Turkey, it's usually arak or ouzo, an anise-infused spirit. (Anise is known to help digestion.) Dozens of these specialties can be enjoyed in one sitting, which lasts several hours and can last until well past midnight, with people enjoying good conversation and listening to music.

Luckily, small plates don't have to be complicated to prepare. Crudités with tahini sauce or labneh alone could qualify as a small plate. So can the Egyptian Fuul Medammes with Tahini in Chapter 17. Of course, each culture has its own concept of which items are served, and some dishes, such as the ones in this chapter, are traditional. Others, however, can be completely up to the chef's interpretation to invent on a whim. In restaurants and in home kitchens, small plates can also help cooks make great use of leftovers.

Authentic Mediterranean Menus

If you're new to making menus, or at least making menus out of small plates, it might seem daunting at first, but there is no need for things to be that way. Let your mood, freshness, and inspiration be your guide. Do a little bit of fridge foraging to see if anything can be repurposed. If so, you've got good small-plate material!

TIP

Here are some starting points for making your own menus:

- » Pick a theme — it could be a country, a few flavors, or a particular ingredient.
- » Make sure that each of the food groups is represented in your menu.
- » Include as many vegetables as possible.
- » Round out the menu with small bowls of spice-dusted nuts, assorted olives, and pickles.

Here are some of my favorites small-plate menus:

- » **Egyptian salatat:**
  - Tahini Sauce, Hummus, and Baba Ghanouj Trio (see recipe in this chapter)
  - Hot pita bread
  - Olives
  - Diced tomato, cucumber, and carrot salad with extra-virgin olive oil and lemon

- » **Provençal picnic:**
  - Fresh Fava Beans with Asparagus and Poached Egg Salad (see recipe in this chapter)
  - Shrimp with Lentils and Garlic (see recipe in this chapter)
  - Fresh bread
  - Sardines with lemon juice
  - Mixed nuts
  - Roasted red bell peppers
  - Goat cheese balls

- » **Greek Islands meze:**
  - Cypriot Imam Biyaldi (Sweet-and-Sour Eggplant; see recipe in this chapter)

- Purslane with Beans, Lemon, Garlic, and Mint (see recipe in this chapter)
- Assorted olives and breads
- Grilled seafood
- Greek cheese plate

>> **Italian antipasti:**

- Broccoli Rabe with Garlic, Extra-Virgin Olive Oil, and Chilies (see recipe in this chapter)
- Cannellini Beans with Artichoke Hearts and Dandelion Greens (see recipe in this chapter)
- Assorted olive, cured meat, and cheese board
- Deviled eggs and *taralli* (crackers), bread, or crostini

>> **Moroccan small plates:**

- Moroccan Vegetable Salad Sampler (see recipe in this chapter)
- Fresh chopped salad
- Preserved lemon, olive, and vegetable bowls
- Fresh bread

The versatile recipes in this section traverse the range of Mediterranean cooking from east to west and can be reworked to fit into lunch, dinner, afternoon aperitif, and brunch schedules as well. These recipes are just a few examples of the many types of small plates that exist.

REMEMBER

Small plates give you license to get creative in the kitchen! Compliment your table of small plates with these easy-to-assemble items:

>> A plate of assorted olives

>> Small bowls of pickled vegetables

>> A cheese board

>> Small bowls of spice-dusted nuts

>> Smoked or preserved fish with a drizzle of lemon juice

>> Cured meats

>> A bread bowl

>> A fresh vegetable and herb platter

>> Deviled eggs

Tahini Sauce, Hummus, and Baba Ghanouj Trio

PREP TIME: ABOUT 15 MIN	COOK TIME: 10 MIN	YIELD: 6 SERVINGS

INGREDIENTS

Tahini Sauce (see the following recipe)

Hummus (see the following recipe)

Baba Ghanouj (see the following recipe)

¼ cup Amy Riolo Selections Extra-Virgin Olive Oil or other good-quality extra-virgin olive oil

¼ teaspoon smoked paprika or Aleppo pepper (optional)

3 cooked whole chickpeas

¼ teaspoon sumac, for garnish (optional)

6 loaves pita bread, for serving

6 celery stalks, trimmed and cut into thirds, for serving (optional)

2 cups cherry tomatoes, for serving (optional)

6 baby or Persian cucumbers, washed and halved lengthwise, for serving (optional)

4 carrots, peeled, trimmed, and cut into sticks, for serving (optional)

2 cups broccoli or cauliflower flowerets, for serving (optional)

1 Spoon the Tahini Sauce, Hummus, and Baba Ghanouj into three equally sized shallow bowls or plates. Smooth the top of each with the back of a clean spoon and make a dent in the center. Drizzle each with olive oil.

2 Sprinkle the Tahini Sauce with smoked paprika or Aleppo pepper, if desired. In the center of the Hummus, place the chickpeas. Sprinkle the top of the Baba Ghanouj with sumac, if desired.

3 Warm the pita bread and place it into a basket or on a plate to serve.

4 On a platter, arrange the celery, tomatoes, cucumbers, carrots, and broccoli or cauliflower in a decorative pattern. Serve.

Tahini Sauce

½ cup tahini

2 teaspoons lemon juice

2 teaspoon vinegar

Dash of cayenne or other hot pepper (optional)

¼ teaspoon salt

1 clove garlic, minced (optional)

¼ cup to ⅓ cup water

1 In a medium bowl, combine the tahini, lemon juice, vinegar, cayenne, salt, and garlic, mixing well with a whisk.

2 Add water, 1 tablespoon at a time, to thin the sauce to a syrupy consistency. The finished product should look like a creamy salad dressing. Cover and store in the refrigerator until needed.

Hummus

2 cups cooked chickpeas, peeled, or rinsed and drained

1 ice cube

2 tablespoons Amy Riolo Selections Extra-Virgin Olive Oil or other good-quality extra-virgin olive oil, divided

Juice of 1 lemon

1 garlic clove

2 tablespoons Tahini Sauce (see the preceding recipe)

Salt to taste

Freshly ground black pepper to taste

Smoked paprika, for garnish

1 In a food processor, place the chickpeas, ice cube, olive oil, lemon juice, garlic, and Tahini Sauce. Process continuously for 2 to 3 minutes, without stopping. Remove the lid and check the consistency. If it's too thick or it hasn't yet formed a paste, add a bit more water. Season with salt and pepper if needed.

(continued)

2 Put the lid back on and continue processing until smooth, about 3 to 5 minutes. Remove the lid, taste again, and adjust the seasonings. Continue processing if needed until a very smooth consistency is achieved.

3 Turn off the processor, remove the lid, and carefully remove the blade. With a plastic spatula, scoop all the hummus into a bowl or a storage container and refrigerate until needed.

Baba Ghanouj

2 medium eggplants

2 tablespoons Tahini Sauce (see the previous recipe)

¼ cup Amy Riolo Selections Extra-Virgin Olive Oil or other good-quality extra-virgin olive oil

Juice of 1 lemon

1 garlic clove, minced

Salt to taste

Freshly ground black pepper to taste

1 Preheat the broiler to 500 degrees. Cover a baking sheet with aluminum foil.

2 Place the eggplants on the baking sheet and prick the eggplant in various places (as you would a baked potato). Place the baking sheet in the oven on the highest rack, closest to the broiler, but without touching it. Broil for a few minutes on each side, watching carefully, until the eggplants are completely charred (like roasted red peppers) in several places. This could take anywhere from 5 to 15 minutes, depending on how close the eggplants are to the broiler. Be sure to watch them carefully and use potholders and large tongs to turn them. The eggplants are done when they're so soft that they shrivel and collapse when held up by tongs. When done, remove from the oven and set the eggplants in a colander over a bowl.

3 As soon as they're cool enough to touch, cut off the tops and remove the skins. Allow the eggplants to drain until all the liquid comes out of them.

4 Take the eggplant pulp out of the colander and transfer it to a large bowl. Mash the pulp with the back of a fork or by squeezing it in your hands until it becomes a mashed consistency.

5 Add the Tahini Sauce, olive oil, lemon juice, and garlic; stir vigorously to combine. Taste and season with salt and pepper, if needed. Cover and store in the refrigerator until needed.

PER SERVING: *Calories 580 (From Fat 325); Fat 36g (Saturated 5g); Cholesterol 0mg; Sodium 477mg; Carbohydrate 56g (Dietary Fiber 15g); Protein 15g.*

A GREAT START

Prior to every meal at restaurants that I worked at in Egypt, every table got this trio served on individual plates along with piping hot bread, olives, and pickles. For me, and many tourists, these dishes themselves were a meal, even though to the locals they were just the beginning. This recipe makes enough servings to keep some extra on hand — or you can double or triple it. Having these three "salads" (as they are called in Egypt) on hand will give you a quick completely healthful and vegan meal in minutes. In addition, each recipe makes a great, portable snack paired with raw vegetables, crackers, or pita bread. I like to take them on my daily walks, picnics, and road trips as well.

The combination of these three recipes in one is a revelation I got from working in restaurants in Egypt. Prior to working in a professional kitchen setting in the Middle East, I made each of these three dishes separately, as do most home cooks. On the first day I worked in Egypt, though, I noticed that they made tahini sauce in large vats because it's the base and required for making hummus, baba ghanouj, and other *meze* as well. This technique is perfect for the home kitchen because it saves time. Even if you don't want to make all three dishes at once, just be sure to prepare the Tahini Sauce often so that you can prepare the Hummus and Baba Ghanouj in just a few minutes.

There is no limit to the number of ways that these dishes can be altered. The Hummus and Baba Ghanouj recipes are pretty standard, but you can use the Tahini Sauce as a salad dressing. Tahini Sauce is also a traditional accompaniment for falafel and fried cauliflower dishes, which are typical in Middle Eastern breakfasts. When I want to ramp up the flavor and make vegetable sides more interesting, I drizzle a little bit of tahini on them. Hummus can become a "bed" for grilled chicken, meat, and seafood. If I have leftover tidbits of any of those, I lay them across the top of the hummus for a new flavor combination. I also recommend trying Baba Ghanouj for breakfast!

Fresh Fava Beans with Asparagus and Poached Egg Salad

PREP TIME: ABOUT 15 MIN	COOK TIME: 15 MIN	YIELD: 4 SERVINGS

INGREDIENTS

16 ounces fresh fava beans

1 bunch asparagus, trimmed and cut on the diagonal in 3-inch slices

1 tablespoon white vinegar

4 large eggs

½ cup chopped, mixed fresh herbs (such as mint, basil, parsley, and dill)

⅓ cup Amy Riolo Selections Extra-Virgin Olive Oil or other good-quality extra-virgin olive oil

3 tablespoons white wine vinegar or juice of 1 lemon

Fleur de sel or unrefined sea salt to taste

Freshly ground pepper to taste

DIRECTIONS

1 Prepare a large pot of salted boiling water and a large bowl of ice water. Drop the fresh fava beans into the boiling water and blanch for 2 to 3 minutes. Carefully remove one bean and test for tenderness. They should taste like a tender, cooked bean when done.

2 Use a slotted spoon to remove the beans, and immerse them in the ice water long enough to cool, about 15 seconds. Drain and place on paper towels to dry, and squeeze them out of their pods.

3 Bring the water back to a boil. Repeat the same process with the asparagus slices, cooking for 3 to 5 minutes. Carefully remove with a slotted spoon, and place in an ice bath to cool.

4 Bring the water back to a boil again. Add the vinegar, and reduce the heat to a simmer.

5 Crack the eggs, one by one, into a ramekin, and carefully slide them into the water. Allow them to cook until the yolks are still soft, about 4 to 6 minutes. (You could also use pre-poached or hardboiled eggs in this step.) When the eggs are finished cooking, carefully remove them with a slotted spoon onto a plate lined with paper towels.

6 Place the beans, asparagus, and herbs on a platter or several small plates. Drizzle with olive oil and white wine vinegar or lemon juice.

7 Place the eggs on top (1 egg per plate or 4 eggs on a large platter) and sprinkle with salt and pepper.

PER SERVING: *Calories 339 (From Fat 209); Fat 23g (Saturated 4g); Cholesterol 212mg; Sodium 273mg; Carbohydrate 21g (Dietary Fiber 6g); Protein 14g.*

TIP: You can use shelled edamame or peas in place of the fava beans if you prefer. You can also substitute frozen beans if you can't find fresh.

TIP: This dish also makes a light and nutrient-dense lunch or dinner on its own.

NOTE: This is a classic Provençal spring dish that's in keeping with the Mediterranean diet. Feel free to swap out your favorite spring beans and peas and mix up the asparagus colors.

VARY IT! For a no-cook, warm-weather option, instead of the egg, top this salad with goat cheese or baked ricotta and some toasted walnuts.

Purslane with Beans, Lemon, Garlic, and Mint

PREP TIME: ABOUT 10 MIN	COOK TIME: NONE	YIELD: 4 SERVINGS

INGREDIENTS

2 bunches fresh purslane, washed, dried, and cut into 2-inch pieces

1 cup cooked cannellini, cranberry beans, or chickpeas

1 clove minced garlic

½ cup chopped fresh mint

¼ cup Amy Riolo Selections Extra-Virgin Olive Oil or other good-quality extra-virgin olive oil

2 tablespoons white balsamic vinegar

Juice of 1 lemon

Sea salt to taste

Freshly ground pepper to taste

DIRECTIONS

1 On a large serving platter, combine the purslane and beans. Set aside.

2 In a small bowl, mix the garlic and mint; mash into a paste with the back of a fork. Set aside.

3 In another small bowl, whisk together the olive oil, vinegar, and lemon juice until emulsified. Taste and season with salt and pepper. Add the garlic and mint mixture and mix well to combine.

4 When ready to serve, whisk the dressing again and pour it over the salad.

PER SERVING: *Calories 209 (From Fat 133); Fat 15g (Saturated 2g); Cholesterol 0mg; Sodium 115mg; Carbohydrate 15g (Dietary Fiber 4g); Protein 5g.*

TIP: Purslane, though not extensively used in the United States, has been a part of the traditional Mediterranean diet since the Minoan civilization used it in ancient Crete. Luckily, purslane is increasingly available in American supermarkets. If you can't find it, substitute the freshest, most nutrient-dense greens you can find, such as dandelion greens, baby kale, baby spinach, or arugula.

NOTE: Purslane is full of omega-3 fatty acids, potassium, vitamin A, vitamin C, magnesium, and iron, just to name a few nutrients. You'll be doing your brain and heart a favor by adding more purslane to your diet.

VARY IT! You can use this recipe as a base formula for whatever beans and greens you have to make a delicious salad. You can also add the ingredients to a skillet and sauté them for a few minutes to serve on top of polenta or bread for a light meal.

Moroccan Vegetable Salad Sampler

PREP TIME: 30 MIN	COOK TIME: 20 MIN	YIELD: 6 SERVINGS

INGREDIENTS

Beets with Cinnamon Salad (see the following recipe)

Potato and Olive Salad (see the following recipe)

Carrot, Orange, and Raisin Salad (see the following recipe)

DIRECTIONS

1 Plate the three salads on three individual dishes or in bowls of a similar size and pattern.

Beets with Cinnamon Salad

4 medium beets, scrubbed, peeled, and cut into 1-inch pieces

1 teaspoon cinnamon

½ teaspoon cumin

½ teaspoon dried ground coriander

¼ cup freshly squeezed lemon juice

3 tablespoons Amy Riolo Selections Extra-Virgin Olive Oil or other good-quality extra-virgin olive oil

½ teaspoon kosher salt

¼ teaspoon freshly ground black pepper

Dash red chili flakes, if desired

1 In a medium saucepan, place the beets and cover with water. Bring to a boil over high heat, reduce the heat to medium, and cook until fork-tender, about 5 to 10 minutes. Drain well.

2 Fill a large bowl three-fourths full of cold water and ice, and place the beets in the ice water. Allow the beets to cool.

3 Drain the beets well, and place them in a large salad bowl. Season with cinnamon, cumin, and coriander. Mix to combine.

4 In a small bowl, pour the lemon juice and slowly add the olive oil while whisking. Add the salt, pepper, and red chili flakes if using. Whisk well to combine. Pour over the beets and serve.

(continued)

Potato and Olive Salad

1 pound golden potatoes, scrubbed, peeled, and cut into 1-inch pieces

1 small red onion, thinly sliced

12 Moroccan olives, or your favorite green variety, pitted and halved

¼ cup freshly squeezed lemon juice

3 tablespoons Amy Riolo Selections Extra-Virgin Olive Oil or other good-quality extra-virgin olive oil

½ teaspoon kosher salt

¼ teaspoon freshly ground black pepper

Pinch of red chili flakes (optional)

1 In a medium saucepan, place the potatoes and cover with water. Bring to a boil over high heat and cook, uncovered, until fork–tender, about 5 to 10 minutes. Drain well and place in a large bowl three–fourths full of cold water and ice. Allow the potatoes to cool, drain well, and place in a large salad bowl. Add the onion and olives, and mix to combine.

2 In a small bowl, pour the lemon juice and slowly add the olive oil while whisking. Add the salt, pepper, and red chili flakes if using. Whisk well to combine. Pour over the salad and serve.

Carrot, Orange, and Raisin Salad

2 cups peeled and shredded carrots

1 navel orange, peeled and cut into segments

¼ cup golden raisins

Juice of 1 orange

Juice of 1 lemon

1 teaspoon orange blossom water

Freshly ground black pepper to taste

1 On a plate, scatter the carrots, making a mound in the middle. Arrange the oranges on top of the carrots. Arrange the raisins around the top.

2 In a small bowl, place the orange juice, lemon juice, orange blossom water, and pepper. Whisk well to combine. Drizzle over the salad, and serve.

PER SERVING: *Calories 288 (From Fat 133); Fat 15g (Saturated 2g); Cholesterol 0mg; Sodium 551mg; Carbohydrate 38g (Dietary Fiber 6g); Protein 4g.*

TIP: You can substitute almost any blanched vegetable for the potato in the Potato and Olive Salad for great results.

VARY IT! Let these recipes be guides and the seasons be your inspiration to create your own Moroccan salads. Try adding leftover beans, cooked grains, chicken, meat, or seafood to "stretch" these salads into a quick yet delicious lunch or entree. The Carrot, Orange, and Raisin Salad could be made the same way with raw beets and apples in place of or in addition to the carrots.

NOTE: I once read a cookbook written by an American that said that Moroccans weren't very into salads. I have the pleasure of leading culinary tours to Morocco every year, and I can assure you that nothing could be farther from the truth. I have enough Moroccan salad recipes to write a book on those alone. In fact, diners at a traditional Moroccan meal are treated to at least seven salads as a matter of course, prior to the entrees. My tour groups are often so impressed by the dazzling colors, fragrant smells, and infinite ways of preparing the vegetables that they're often filled up before their main course arrives. From a health perspective, this is fantastic because they're getting their fill (literally) of nutrient-rich produce. Moroccans use both cooked and raw vegetables in salads, and they serve them together.

Broccoli Rabe with Garlic, Extra–Virgin Olive Oil, and Chilies

PREP TIME: ABOUT 5 MIN	COOK TIME: 5 MIN	YIELD: 4 SERVINGS

INGREDIENTS

2 bunches fresh broccoli rabe, ½ inch of ends trimmed

3 tablespoons Amy Riolo Selections Extra-Virgin Olive Oil or other good-quality extra-virgin olive oil, divided

¼ teaspoon unrefined sea salt

⅛ teaspoon freshly ground black pepper

¼ teaspoon red chile flakes

4 cloves garlic, minced

DIRECTIONS

1 Prepare a large pot of salted boiling water and a large bowl of ice water. Drop the broccoli rabe into the boiling water and blanch for 2 minutes. Remove and immerse in the ice water long enough to cool, about 15 seconds. Drain and place on paper towels to dry.

2 In a large, wide skillet, add 2 tablespoons of the olive oil and warm over medium heat. Add the broccoli rabe and, using tongs, turn to coat in the oil. Season with salt, pepper, and crushed red chile flakes.

3 Continue cooking and turning until the broccoli rabe is golden but still retains a bit of its crunch, about 5 minutes.

4 Add the garlic and sauté until the garlic begins to release its aroma, about 1 minute. Drizzle with remaining 1 tablespoon of olive oil and serve warm.

PER SERVING: *Calories 98 (From Fat 92); Fat 10g (Saturated 1g); Cholesterol 0mg; Sodium 153mg; Carbohydrate 2g (Dietary Fiber 1g); Protein 1g.*

TIP: This delicious dish is loaded with antioxidants and anti-inflammatories that will help keep you looking and feeling great. Use it as a side dish for grilled, roasted, or pan-fried poultry and seafood if you like.

NOTE: You can toss this recipe in with cooked spaghetti, rice, or other grains for a complete meal.

VARY IT! This is a classic Calabrian method of cooking most green vegetables. Artichokes, asparagus, dandelion greens, spinach, kale, Swiss chard, cabbage, regular broccoli, cauliflower, Brussels sprouts, and peppers can all be prepared using this technique for excellent health-boosting and flavor-enhancing results. With the softer greens, you can even skip the blanching step and just begin by sautéing the greens in the olive oil. If you have leftovers, you can add them to a soup or puree them to use as a "bed" for poultry or seafood. Or add a little bit of stock to the puree to make a homemade soup.

Cannellini Beans with Artichoke Hearts and Dandelion Greens

PREP TIME: ABOUT 10 MIN	COOK TIME: 5 MIN	YIELD: 4 SERVINGS

INGREDIENTS

¼ cup Amy Riolo Selections Extra-Virgin Olive Oil or other good-quality extra-virgin olive oil, divided

2 bunches fresh dandelion greens, chopped

1 cup cooked cannellini beans

2 cups cooked artichoke hearts

½ cup chopped fresh basil, plus 4 leaves for garnish

2 cloves garlic, minced

Sea salt to taste

Freshly ground black pepper to taste

2 tablespoons white balsamic vinegar

DIRECTIONS

1 In a large, wide skillet, place 2 tablespoons of the oil and warm over medium heat.

2 Add the dandelion greens and stir with a wooden spoon, cooking, uncovered, until tender and wilted, about 3 minutes. Add the beans, artichoke hearts, basil, and garlic, and cook together for a few minutes. Taste and season with salt and pepper.

3 When ready to serve, drizzle with the remaining 2 tablespoons of olive oil and the vinegar and toss to combine. Transfer to a platter or small plates, garnish with basil leaves, and serve warm.

PER SERVING: *Calories 248 (From Fat 129); Fat 14g (Saturated 2g); Cholesterol 0mg; Sodium 259mg; Carbohydrate 26g (Dietary Fiber 13g); Protein 7g.*

TIP: If you can't find dandelion greens, you can use chicory or Swiss chard instead. You can replace the cannellini beans with cranberry beans or chickpeas, too.

VARY IT! Puree the beans prior to serving and add the cooked greens and artichokes to the top. Alternately, heat some stock and cook all three ingredients in it — perhaps adding in a bit of wheatberries, rice, or barley for a delicious and unique *minestra*, which is an Italian soup made with various combinations of legumes, grains, and vegetables.

NOTE: Beans and greens of all stripes and cooking preparations are popular in my ancestral homeland of Southern Italy, as well as around the Mediterranean. Enjoying a meal based around a dish like this daily is a great idea. I love dandelion greens because their taste reminds me of my childhood. They also provide more than five times the recommended daily value of vitamin K, which strengthens bones and may also play a role in fighting Alzheimer's disease. Dandelion greens also give the body 112 percent of the daily minimum requirement of vitamin A as an antioxidant carotenoid, which is needed for the skin, mucus membranes, and vision. There are so many additional nutrients to list — in fact, their ancient Latin name meant "official disease remedy." Learning to love them in lots of preparations will benefit you immensely.

Cypriot Imam Biyaldi (Sweet-and-Sour Eggplant)

PREP TIME: ABOUT 10 MIN	COOK TIME: 1 HR 10 MIN	YIELD: 8 SERVINGS

INGREDIENTS

8 small or Japanese-style eggplants, washed and dried

¼ cup unrefined sea salt

3 cups Amy Riolo Selections Extra-Virgin Olive Oil or other good-quality extra-virgin olive oil, divided

2 medium yellow onions, sliced

1 tablespoon sugar

2 garlic cloves, diced

1 tablespoon tomato paste, divided

1½ cups tomato puree

½ cup finely chopped fresh parsley

2 tablespoons finely chopped fresh basil leaves

Salt to taste

Freshly ground black pepper to taste

½ cup feta or graviera cheese, for garnish (optional)

DIRECTIONS

1 Remove the stems from the eggplants, and slice the eggplants in half lengthwise. Place the eggplants, cut side up, on a large baking sheet, and sprinkle with the ¼ cup of sea salt. Allow to stand for at least 1 hour. Rinse off the salt and dry well. Set aside.

2 In a large, wide skillet with at least 3-inch-high sides, warm 2½ cups of the olive oil over medium-high heat. Bring the oil to a temperature of approximately 375 degrees.

3 Carefully lower the eggplants into the oil and fry them with the cut side facing down until they've become soft and slightly golden, about 3 to 4 minutes, turning if necessary.

4 Line a baking sheet with paper towels and, using a slotted spoon, transfer the eggplants to the baking sheet, cut side facing down, in order to absorb as much olive oil as possible. Continue with the remaining eggplant slices.

5 When you're finished frying the eggplants, set aside the hot pan to cool.

6 In another large skillet heat the remaining ¼ cup of olive oil and sauté the onion over medium-low heat, stirring often, until it's very soft and translucent, about 5 to 10 minutes.

7 Add the garlic and sauté until it releases its aroma, about 1 minute.

8 Add the sugar and stir. Reduce the heat to low and continue to cook, mixing every now and then, until they begin to caramelize, about 15 to 20 minutes.

9 Make a small dent in the bottom of the pan by moving the onions to the side. Add the tomato paste with a wooden spoon, and stir while allowing it to caramelize for a moment on its own.

10 Next add the tomato puree, parsley, salt, and pepper. Increase the heat to high and bring to a boil. Reduce the heat to medium-low, cover with the lid ajar, and simmer until the sauce reduces by half, about 10 to 20 minutes. Remove from the heat and let it cool for a while.

11 Preheat the oven to 425 degrees.

12 Scoop some flesh out of the eggplant to make room for the filling. Add the eggplant pulp to the filling mixture and spoon it inside the eggplant. Put the eggplants in a large baking dish or on a baking sheet with the cut side facing up. Add the crumbled feta or graviera cheese on top. Drizzle with remaining ¼ cup olive oil.

13 Bake until golden, about 30 minutes. Allow to cool for 30 minutes and top with basil before serving slightly warm or at room temperature.

PER SERVING: *Calories 221 (From Fat 119); Fat 13g (Saturated 3g); Cholesterol 8mg; Sodium 829mg; Carbohydrate 25g (Dietary Fiber 5g); Protein 4g.*

TIP: This is the most time-consuming of all the small-plate recipes in this chapter, but it's definitely worth it. This recipe is my mother's favorite, and it tastes even better the next day, so don't be afraid to make extra.

VARY IT! You don't need to take the extra step of baking the eggplant with cheese in the oven. Some people finish the eggplants by adding them in to the tomato sauce and letting them simmer for 10 to 15 minutes until they're very tender and a stewlike consistency is achieved. Note that there are many variations on this dish. Some people also add raisins and pine nuts to the dish, so don't be afraid to change it up!

LEGEND HAS IT . . .

The name *Imam Biyaldi* is a Turkish term that means that the imam fainted, and the reasons for this reaction are many, depending on who tells the story of the recipe. Both Greeks and Turks make the recipe nowadays, and it's part of the traditional Greek Ladera dishes made with olive oil during Lent, when people abstain from eating animal fats. Note that, during Lent, the cheese would not be added to this recipe. In Turkey, the same category of dishes exist (even though nowadays they aren't reserved for fasting Orthodox Christians) and are called *zeytinyağlılar* (zay-*tin* yah-*luh*-lar), which means "those with olive oil." In Turkey, the term refers to cooked vegetables that are dressed with olive oil and served cold.

Regardless, both countries' olive-oil-based recipes offer countless sources of inspiration for seekers of delicious Mediterranean diet-friendly recipes. Some say this recipe got its name because an imam fainted after tasting his wife's delicious eggplant dish. In Cyprus, they say that the wife was the daughter of a Greek olive oil merchant, which is why she used so much oil in the recipes. Others say that the imam fainted when he found out the cost of the oil, and so on. . . . I hope you'll swoon over the flavor and not mind the occasional splurge on extra-virgin olive oil.

Shrimp with Lentils and Garlic

PREP TIME: ABOUT 10 MIN	COOK TIME: 5 MIN	YIELD: 6 SERVINGS

INGREDIENTS

2 tablespoons Amy Riolo Selections Extra-Virgin Olive Oil or other good-quality extra-virgin olive oil, divided

1½ pounds shrimp, peeled and deveined

3 cloves garlic, sliced

1 teaspoon herbes de Provence or your favorite dried herbs or spices

¼ teaspoon unrefined sea salt

1 lemon, halved, divided

1 cup cooked green or brown lentils

1 lemon, quartered

DIRECTIONS

1 In a large skillet, warm 1 tablespoon of the olive oil over medium-high heat. After the olive oil begins to release its aroma, about 1 minute, add the shrimp, garlic, herbes de Provence, and salt. Cook until the shrimp are bright pink and cooked through, about 2 to 3 minutes per side. Squeeze the juice of half of a lemon on top and remove from the heat.

2 If the lentils are cold, reheat them and place on plate. Top with the shrimp. Squeeze the juice of the other lemon half over top, and drizzle with the remaining 1 tablespoon of olive oil. Place the lemon quarters around the plate.

PER SERVING: *Calories 202 (From Fat 59); Fat 7g (Saturated 1g); Cholesterol 172mg; Sodium 266mg; Carbohydrate 9g (Dietary Fiber 3g); Protein 26g.*

TIP: Be sure to cook the shrimp just until done — overcooking makes them tough. Any size shrimp works in this recipe. Serve with toasted bread rubbed with garlic and a green salad for a complete meal.

NOTE: I've tasted varieties of this dish in many coastal Mediterranean cities. Note that the same dish could be served with just shrimp alone. Instead of serving the lentils whole, you can puree them and use them as a smooth "bed" for the shrimp. I love this dish because it helps coax people who love shrimp into eating more lentils, an ingredient that is at the core of the Mediterranean diet.

VARY IT! Scallops or small pieces of fish also work in this recipe. You could also sauté vegetables, such as bright bell peppers, to place on top.

Snacking in the Mediterranean

Snacking is part of the Mediterranean lifestyle just as it is in the United States, but less emphasis is placed on it. People tend to snack either on street foods if they aren't home or on healthful combinations that are simply meant to carry them from one meal to another.

In most family and rural settings, snacks are less important because the main meals are so full of satisfying and nutrient-dense foods that people don't need to snack between meals.

TIP

If you do find yourself hungry in between meals, try some of these Mediterranean options:

>> Almonds, walnuts, or cooked chickpeas roasted or dry pan-fried with your favorite spice mix

>> Watermelon seeds, lupini seeds, sunflower seeds, or *pepitas* (pumpkin seeds)

>> Dried dates

>> No-sugar-added dried figs, apricots, and other fruits

>> A serving of Greek yogurt with a teaspoon of extra-virgin olive oil or honey

>> A piece of fresh fruit and a handful of almonds

TIP

Most dishes in this chapter (especially the salads and the Tahini Sauce, Hummus, and Baba Ghanouj Trio) make wonderful snacks when you're on the go. Try to keep these items on hand and take them with you if you know you'll have to go a long time between meals.

Chapter **19**

Base Recipes and Main Courses

This chapter includes beloved Mediterranean recipes that beautifully exemplify the nutritious diet. Each recipe is versatile, relatively easy to make, and lesser known in the United States. In this chapter, I explain the role that the ingredients and dishes play in the typical Mediterranean meal and offer tips and tricks to enjoying them easily at home.

Base Recipes for Any Mediterranean Meal

The simple recipes in this section are the backbone of the Mediterranean kitchen. Replacing store-bought ingredients with these homemade staple ingredients will improve the overall taste of your dishes and save you time and money, while cutting excess sodium, calories, and preservatives from your meals.

Whenever I prepare these recipes, I make them in large quantities and store them. In fact, every recipe in this chapter can be prepared and then frozen for later use. With roasted peppers, stocks, beans, lentils, and fresh bread crumbs in your freezer, you'll always be prepared to whip up healthful, inexpensive soups, pastas, salads, and purees in no time!

In my Mediterranean Diet Made Easy Cooking Class series, I had my students make these recipes in the very first class and then use them to cook with on the second day. I even taught teenagers this method — and if they can do it, so can you!

TIP

If for some reason you absolutely have to use packaged and processed pantry items instead of these, be sure to read the labels to get the lowest amounts of unwanted ingredients possible. Otherwise, try swapping those ingredients out for better options. I would rather use plain water with herbs and/or spices than have to buy a packaged stock that is full of sodium and ingredients that I can't pronounce.

Roasted Red Peppers

PREP TIME: ABOUT 5 MIN	COOK TIME: 40 MIN	YIELD: 4 SERVINGS

INGREDIENTS

4 red bell peppers

1 tablespoon Amy Riolo Selections Extra-Virgin Olive Oil or other good-quality extra-virgin olive oil

DIRECTIONS

1 Preheat the oven to 500 degrees.

2 On a baking sheet, place the whole bell peppers. Place in the oven until the skins are wrinkled and the peppers are charred, about 30 to 40 minutes, being sure to turn them each time a side is charred (approximately twice during cooking).

3 Remove from the oven and cover tightly with aluminum foil to create steam. Set aside.

4 When peppers are cool enough to handle, after about 30 minutes, cut into quarters, peel off the skin, and remove the seeds. Add to your favorite recipe or, if not eating immediately, place the pepper pieces in a jar, cover with olive oil for additional flavor and nutrition, and seal with a lid; refrigerate up to 2 weeks. Drain the oil from the peppers before using and reserve in the refrigerator for another use.

PER SERVING: *Calories 81 (From Fat 35); Fat 4g (Saturated 1g); Cholesterol 0mg; Sodium 7mg; Carbohydrate 10g (Dietary Fiber 3g); Protein 2g.*

TIP: If you'd rather freeze the peppers for later use, place the pieces in a resealable plastic bag and freeze up to 1 month.

Dried Beans

| PREP TIME: 1 HR | COOK TIME: 30 MIN | YIELD: 8 SERVINGS |

INGREDIENTS

1 cup dried beans (any variety)

¼ teaspoon unrefined sea salt

DIRECTIONS

1 Place the beans in a stockpot and cover with cold water; leave to soak overnight. (If you're short on time, place the beans in a stockpot, cover with boiling water, and leave to soak for 1 hour instead.)

2 Drain the soaked beans and place them in a saucepan. Add the salt, cover the beans with water, and bring to a boil over high heat.

3 Reduce the heat to medium-low, cover, and let cook until the beans are tender, about 25 to 50 minutes. (It may take longer depending on the size of the beans.)

4 Drain and cool. If not using right away, store in an airtight container in the refrigerator for up to 1 week.

PER SERVING: *Calories 83 (From Fat 2); Fat 0g (Saturated 0g); Cholesterol 0mg; Sodium 215mg; Carbohydrate 15g (Dietary Fiber 4g); Protein 6g.*

Braised Cannellini Beans

PREP TIME: ABOUT 5 MIN PLUS 8 HR TO OVERNIGHT FOR SOAKING	COOK TIME: 40 MIN	YIELD: 8 SERVINGS

INGREDIENTS

1 cup dried cannellini beans

4 rosemary sprigs, divided

1 tablespoon Amy Riolo Selections Extra-Virgin Olive Oil or other good-quality extra-virgin olive oil

¼ teaspoon unrefined sea salt

DIRECTIONS

1 In a large bowl, add the cannellini beans and enough cold water to cover them by 4 inches. Let soak in a cool place or in the refrigerator for at least 8 hours or overnight.

2 Drain the beans and transfer them to a 2-quart saucepan. Pour in enough water to cover by 1 inch, and drop in 2 rosemary sprigs. Bring the water to a boil, and then lower the heat so the water is barely at a simmer. Cook until the beans are tender but not mushy, with just enough liquid to cover them, about 30 to 40 minutes. (If necessary, add more water, 1 tablespoon at a time, to keep the beans covered as they simmer.)

3 Remove the beans from the heat and gently stir in the olive oil, sea salt, and the remaining 2 rosemary sprigs. Let the beans stand to cool and absorb the cooking liquid. The end result should be tender beans with a creamy consistency in just enough liquid to coat them. If you're not using them right away, store the beans in an airtight container in the refrigerator up to 1 week.

PER SERVING: *Calories 92 (From Fat 18); Fat 2g (Saturated 0g); Cholesterol 0mg; Sodium 76mg; Carbohydrate 14g (Dietary Fiber 5g); Protein 5g.*

Lentils

PREP TIME: ABOUT 5 MIN | **COOK TIME: 30 MIN** | **YIELD: 6 SERVINGS**

INGREDIENTS

1 cup dried lentils (any variety)

¼ teaspoon unrefined sea salt

¼ teaspoon freshly ground black pepper

1 bay leaf

DIRECTIONS

1 Rinse the lentils in a colander.

2 In a saucepan, place the lentils and add enough water to cover them twice (you should have twice as much water as lentils). Add the sea salt, pepper, and bay leaf. Bring to a boil over high heat. Then reduce the heat to low and simmer, uncovered, until the lentils are tender, about 5 to 30 minutes depending on the variety. (Red lentils are the quickest-cooking variety, followed by green and brown, and then black.)

3 If you're not using them right away, store cooked lentils in an airtight container in the refrigerator up to 1 week.

PER SERVING: *Calories 113 (From Fat 3); Fat 0g (Saturated 0g); Cholesterol 0mg; Sodium 99mg; Carbohydrate 19g (Dietary Fiber 10g); Protein 8g.*

Homemade Vegetable Stock

PREP TIME: ABOUT 5 MIN	COOK TIME: 30 MIN	YIELD: 8 SERVINGS

INGREDIENTS

1 onion, halved (not peeled)

1 carrot, trimmed and halved

1 stalk celery, trimmed and halved (can include leaves, if desired)

4 ounces cherry tomatoes

4 sprigs fresh basil, with stems

1 small bunch fresh flat-leaf parsley, with stems

½ teaspoon salt

DIRECTIONS

1 In a large stock pot, place the onion, carrot, celery, tomatoes, basil, and parsley. Cover with 16 cups water. Bring to a boil over high heat. Then reduce the heat to medium–low. Add the salt and simmer, uncovered, for 30 minutes.

2 Drain the stock, reserving the liquid. Discard the rest. If you're not using it right away, allow to cool and then store in the refrigerator or freezer.

PER SERVING: *Calories 11 (From Fat 0); Fat 0g (Saturated 0g); Cholesterol 0mg; Sodium 145mg; Carbohydrate 2g (Dietary Fiber 0g); Protein 1g.*

Homemade Seafood Stock

PREP TIME: ABOUT 15 MIN	COOK TIME: 30 MIN	YIELD: 8 SERVINGS

INGREDIENTS

1 onion, halved (not peeled)

1 carrot, trimmed, and halved

1 stalk celery, halved

Shells from 2 pounds shrimp

½ teaspoon salt

1 dried bay leaf

1 tablespoon whole black peppercorns

DIRECTIONS

1 In a large stock pot, place the onion, carrot, celery, and shrimp shells. Cover with 16 cups water. Bring to a boil over high heat. Then reduce the heat to medium-low.

2 Skim off the residue that forms on top of the stock and discard. Add the salt, bay leaf, and peppercorns. Simmer, uncovered, for about 30 minutes.

3 Drain the stock, reserving the liquid. Discard the rest. If you're not using it right away, allow to cool, and then store in the refrigerator or freezer.

PER SERVING: *Calories 39 (From Fat 7); Fat 1g (Saturated 0g); Cholesterol 0mg; Sodium 145mg; Carbohydrate 1g (Dietary Fiber 0g); Protein 5g.*

Homemade Chicken Stock

PREP TIME: ABOUT 5 MIN	COOK TIME: 40 MIN	YIELD: 8 SERVINGS

INGREDIENTS

1 medium onion, halved (not peeled)

1 medium carrot, trimmed and halved

1 medium stalk celery, halved

1¼ pounds chicken bones or carcass from cooked chicken

1 teaspoon whole black peppercorns

1 dried bay leaf

½ teaspoon salt

DIRECTIONS

1 In a large stock pot, place the onion, carrot, celery, chicken bones, peppercorns, and bay leaf. Cover with 16 cups water. Bring to a boil over high heat. Then reduce the heat to medium-low.

2 Skim off the residue that forms on top of the stock and discard. Add the salt and simmer, uncovered, for 40 minutes.

3 Drain the stock, reserving the liquid. Discard the rest. If you're not using it right away, allow to cool, and then store in the refrigerator or freezer.

PER SERVING: *Calories 39 (From Fat 11); Fat 1g (Saturated 0g); Cholesterol 0mg; Sodium 145mg; Carbohydrate 1g (Dietary Fiber 0g); Protein 5g.*

Mediterranean Main Courses

This section contains versatile Mediterranean mains that will add color, flavor, and nutrition to your repertoire. Each of these dishes can be altered in numerous ways so you can get more recipes and ideas out of them. These recipes also span the Mediterranean and can be considered meals in themselves — no need for salads or sides.

Tajine Djaj bil Couscous (Moroccan Chicken, Almond, and Olive Tajine with Couscous)

PREP TIME: 30 MIN	COOK TIME: 1 HR	YIELD: 8 SERVINGS

INGREDIENTS

3 tablespoons Amy Riolo Selections Extra-Virgin Olive Oil or other good-quality extra-virgin olive oil, divided

3 pounds chicken thighs and legs with skin and bones

1 medium onion, diced

1 teaspoon ground cinnamon

1 teaspoon cardamom pods

½ teaspoon freshly ground black pepper

1 teaspoon cumin

1½ teaspoons saffron, divided

2 cups reduced-sodium chicken stock

1 cup blanched almonds, divided

1 cup green olives, rinsed

2 cups couscous

Salt, to taste

DIRECTIONS

1 In a large skillet, warm 2 tablespoons of the oil over medium-high heat.

2 Add the chicken pieces and sauté until golden brown in color on each side, about 3 minutes per side. Remove from the pan and set aside.

3 To the same skillet, add the onions, cinnamon, cardamom, black pepper, cumin, and ½ teaspoon of the saffron. Stir and sauté until the onions are tender, about 10 minutes.

4 Return the chicken to the skillet and add just enough stock to cover. Add the blanched almonds and olives. Stir and lower the heat to medium-low. Cover and simmer until the chicken is cooked through and the almonds are tender, about 45 minutes.

5 While the chicken is simmering, prepare the couscous. In a medium saucepan with a lid, bring 2 cups water and the remaining 1 teaspoon of saffron to a boil, uncovered. When the water is boiling, remove the pan from the heat and add the couscous. Mix well, cover the pan with the lid, and let stand for 5 to 10 minutes. Remove the lid and add the remaining 1 tablespoon of olive oil. Stir, add the salt, and fluff with a fork.

6 Spoon the couscous onto a large serving platter. Remove the cardamom pods from the chicken tajine and arrange the chicken on top of the couscous.

PER SERVING: *Calories 394 (From Fat 176); Fat 20g (Saturated 3g); Cholesterol 13mg; Sodium 301mg; Carbohydrate 42g (Dietary Fiber 5g); Protein 15g.*

Agnello al Forno in Pignata (Southern Italian Lamb Stew)

PREP TIME: ABOUT 15 MIN | **COOK TIME: 3 HR 20 MIN** | **YIELD: 6 SERVINGS**

INGREDIENTS

¼ cup Amy Riolo Selections Extra-Virgin Olive Oil or other good-quality extra-virgin olive oil

1 large yellow onion, peeled and diced

2 carrots, peeled and diced

1 stalk celery, diced

6 cloves garlic, sliced

2½ pounds lamb shoulder meat cubes (from the thigh or shoulder), about 1½-inch each

½ cup dry white wine

⅛ teaspoon unrefined sea salt

1 bay leaf

4 cups Homemade Chicken Stock (see recipe earlier in this chapter), reduced-sodium chicken stock, or water

4 red bell peppers, cored and cut into 1-inch pieces

1 cup peeled, crushed tomatoes

1 teaspoon crushed red chile flakes, chile powder, or chile paste

DIRECTIONS

1 Preheat the oven to 350 degrees.

2 In a large, heavy-bottomed, ovenproof saucepan or Dutch, place the olive oil and warm over medium-high heat.

3 Add the onions, carrots, and celery, and turn to coat in the oil. Reduce the heat to medium-low and sauté the vegetables until tender, about 10 minutes. Add the garlic, stir, and cook until it releases its aroma, about 1 minute.

4 Add the lamb meat and cook, turning, until browned on all sides, about 3 to 5 minutes. Add the wine and increase the heat to high. When liquid is almost completely evaporated, after about 10 minutes, season with salt. Add the bay leaf and stock or water and bring to a boil. Stir, reduce the heat to low, cover, and place in the oven for 2 hours, stirring occasionally.

5 Carefully remove the pan from the oven and use oven mitts to remove the lid. Add the peppers, tomatoes, and chile. Stir and cover. Cook until the meat is very tender, about 1 hour. Remove the bay leaf, if desired, and serve.

PER SERVING: *Calories 365 (From Fat 185); Fat 21g (Saturated 5g); Cholesterol 76mg; Sodium 188mg; Carbohydrate 16g (Dietary Fiber 3g); Protein 27g.*

NOTE: A *pignata* is a cylindrical terra-cotta pot used to make stews in the Calabria and some other regions of Southern Italy. Traditionally, the stews would cook in the hearth slowly while bread and other items were being made. The shape of a *pignata* (with two handles on the sides) made them easy to transport to homes or to the fields. There is a strong tradition of cooking with earthenware throughout the Mediterranean, which is healthful and delicious. Nowadays, many of these dishes are being made in Dutch ovens or pressure cookers on the stovetop.

VARY IT! You can use any kind of meat — goat, chicken, beef, veal, and so on — in place of the lamb and cook it until the desired amount of doneness is achieved.

Pollo alla Amontillado con Patatas Arrugadas y Pico Mahon (Spanish Sherry Chicken with Potatoes in Mojo Picón Sauce)

PREP TIME: ABOUT 10 MIN	COOK TIME: 15 MIN	YIELD: 4 SERVINGS

INGREDIENTS

¾ cup Amy Riolo Selections Extra-Virgin Olive Oil or other good-quality extra-virgin olive oil, divided

1 head garlic, separated into individual cloves (skin left on)

4 chicken breasts, halved, width-wise and each half cut into 3 pieces

¼ teaspoon unrefined sea salt

⅛ teaspoon freshly ground black pepper

1 cup dry sherry

1 pound of small fingerling or other baby potatoes

½ cup plus ½ teaspoon salt, divided

¼ cup drained roasted red peppers

2 teaspoons sweet paprika

1 teaspoon ground cumin

¼ cup white wine vinegar

¼ cup chopped fresh cilantro, for garnish

DIRECTIONS

1 In a large, wide skillet, place ¼ cup of the oil, and warm over medium–high heat.

2 Add the garlic cloves and cook, turning, until they release their aroma and turn golden and soft, 3 or 4 minutes. Using tongs, carefully remove the garlic cloves and set them on a platter.

3 Add the chicken to the oil and season with sea salt and pepper. Allow to cook until golden on each side, about 3 to 4 minutes, and turn. Continue to cook and turn occasionally until the chicken is golden.

4 Increase the heat to high and carefully pour the sherry over the chicken. Stir and cover with a lid. Reduce the heat to medium–low and cook until the sherry is almost evaporated and the chicken is cooked to 165 degrees, about 5 to 10 minutes. Leave covered and set aside.

5 In a large pot, place the potatoes and cover with water. Add ½ cup of the salt. Bring to a boil over high heat, uncovered. Then reduce the heat to medium. Continue cooking until the potatoes are fork tender, about 10 minutes.

6 Drain the potatoes without turning off the heat and return them to the pot. Put the pot back on top of the same burner and continue to cook with the heat off until they dry and obtain a wrinkled appearance, about 2 minutes.

(continued)

7 To make the sauce, peel the reserved garlic and put it into a high-speed blender with the roasted red peppers, paprika, and cumin to create a paste. Add the remaining ½ cup of olive oil, vinegar, and the remaining ½ teaspoon of salt. Blend on high speed until the ingredients are incorporated, 3 to 4 minutes. Taste and adjust the seasonings as needed.

8 To serve, pour half of the sauce in the center of a platter. Add the chicken pieces and potatoes. Drizzle the remaining sauce over the top. Garnish with fresh cilantro, if desired, and serve.

PER SERVING: *Calories 791 (From Fat 431); Fat 48g (Saturated 7g); Cholesterol 151mg; Sodium 989mg; Carbohydrate 25g (Dietary Fiber 2g); Protein 52g.*

NOTE: These potatoes are called "wrinkly potatoes" in Spanish because of the salt bath that they cook in.

TIP: Make extra chicken and sauce to use in different ways throughout the week.

NOTE: This recipe is actually a combination of two different classic Spanish dishes. Normally, the chicken with the sherry sauce is not always served with the "wrinkly" potatoes and mojo picón sauce, but I think they're fabulous together and the flavors really play well off each other. Mojo is actually a type of sauce that originated in the Canary Islands where both green and red varieties are popular.

VARY IT! Turkey and duck meat work well instead of the chicken, and broccoli tastes great cooked in the same way as the potatoes.

Pasta al Forno con Melanzane e Caciocavallo (Baked Pasta with Eggplant and Caciocavallo)

PREP TIME: ABOUT 20 MIN PLUS 1 HR FOR RESTING	COOK TIME: 1 HR	YIELD: 8 SERVINGS

INGREDIENTS

2 medium eggplants

¼ cup unrefined sea salt

¼ cup plus 3 tablespoons plus 1 teaspoon Amy Riolo Selections Extra-Virgin Olive Oil or other good-quality extra-virgin olive oil, divided

1 garlic clove, sliced

One 14.5-ounce can crushed plum tomatoes

1 handful fresh basil leaves, chopped

¼ teaspoon freshly ground black pepper

1 pound rigatoni or penne pasta

¼ pound caciocavallo cheese, or other semiaged cow milk cheese, thinly sliced

3 hardboiled eggs, peeled and diced

1 cup pecorino cheese

DIRECTIONS

1 Cut the stem off of the eggplants and cut them into large cubes. Place them in a colander and cover with the salt. Let stand to draw the moisture out of the eggplant cubes, about 1 hour.

2 In a large saucepan, add 2 tablespoons of the extra-virgin olive oil and warm over medium heat. Add the garlic, and stir with a wooden spoon. The minute that the garlic releases its aroma (prior to turning color), add the plum tomatoes and stir with a wooden spoon. Add the basil and salt and pepper to taste. Bring the sauce to a boil over high heat. Cover, and reduce the heat to low. Simmer for 10 minutes. Carefully remove the lid and stir, being sure to incorporate the bits from the sides of the pan. Taste and adjust the seasoning if necessary.

3 Bring a large pot of water to a boil over high heat, and add 1 teaspoon of salt. Add the pasta, stir, lower the heat to medium-low, and cook until very al dente (meaning extra firm, because it will cook again in the oven), about 6 minutes.

4 While the pasta is cooking, rinse off the reserved eggplant to get rid of the salt and juice residue and dry them well.

(continued)

5 In a large, wide skillet, place 2 tablespoons of the olive oil and warm over medium-high heat. Carefully add the eggplant, working in batches if necessary so there is only one even layer over the bottom. Turn the eggplant and cook until golden and tender, about 5 minutes.

6 In the meantime, drain the pasta when it's ready and run it under cold water for 1 minute to stop further cooking.

7 Preheat the oven to 375 degrees. Lightly oil a 9-x-13-inch ceramic or glass baking dish.

8 Take a ladle of tomato sauce and stir it into the pasta. Pour the pasta into the baking dish. Cover the pasta with the caciocavallo cheese and sprinkle the egg pieces over the top. Cover with the eggplant slices and the remaining sauce. Top by evenly distributing the pecorino cheese and drizzle the remaining 3 tablespoons of extra-virgin olive oil over the top.

9 Bake until golden and crispy on top, about 15 minutes. Remove and allow to cool slightly before serving.

PER SERVING: *Calories 364 (From Fat 204); Fat 23g (Saturated 7g); Cholesterol 104mg; Sodium 689mg; Carbohydrate 26g (Dietary Fiber 3g); Protein 15g.*

TIP: This dish is great to make in advance and is often enjoyed at buffets. It's a meal in itself, and it makes an easy and impressive lunch or dinner with a simple green salad.

NOTE: Calabrians loved baked pasta dishes — this one combines beloved eggplant with the region's prized Caciocavallo Silano cheese. Even hard-boiled eggs (another regional touch) get added into the mix.

VARY IT! You can use different types of pasta and cheese to come up with your own favorite combination of this classic dish. You can also add in leftover bits of vegetables and meat if you like.

Yachni (Greek Tomato and Vegetable Stew)

PREP TIME: ABOUT 15 MIN	COOK TIME: 1 HR 35 MIN	YIELD: 4 SERVINGS

INGREDIENTS

2 tablespoons Amy Riolo Selections Extra-Virgin Olive Oil or other good-quality extra-virgin olive oil

1 yellow onion, diced

1½ pounds stew meat

2 cups tomato puree or crushed tomatoes

1 bay leaf

½ pound green beans, trimmed, or lima beans

1 eggplant, chopped into 2-inch cubes (optional)

1 cup peas (optional)

½ pound okra, tops trimmed and sliced into rounds (optional)

3 potatoes, peeled and cubed (optional)

1 head cauliflower, cut flowerets only (optional)

1 cup cooked dried beans (optional)

1 teaspoon sea salt

¼ teaspoon freshly ground pepper

DIRECTIONS

1 In a large saucepan, warm the olive oil over medium heat. Add the onion and meat, and sauté until brown, about 5 minutes.

2 Add the tomatoes and enough water to cover the meat. Add the bay leaf. Increase the heat to high and bring to a boil. Reduce the heat to low, cover, and simmer for 1 hour.

3 Add the green beans, eggplant, peas, okra, potatoes, cauliflower, beans, salt, and pepper, and stir. Continue to cook until tender, about 30 minutes. Taste and adjust the seasoning if desired.

PER SERVING: *Calories 506 (From Fat 219); Fat 24g (Saturated 7g); Cholesterol 95mg; Sodium 743mg; Carbohydrate 29g (Dietary Fiber 9g); Protein 55g.*

Pesce alla Siciliana con Verdure al Forno (Roasted Sicilian–Style Fish with Vegetables)

PREP TIME: ABOUT 15 MIN | **COOK TIME: 40 MIN** | **YIELD: 4 SERVINGS**

INGREDIENTS

1 pound tuna, snapper, bass, or swordfish or other fish fillets, cut into four 4-ounce pieces

3 tablespoons Amy Riolo Selections Extra-Virgin Olive Oil or other good-quality extra-virgin olive oil, plus more as needed

1 medium yellow onion, finely chopped

1 celery heart, finely chopped

1 carrot, peeled and finely chopped

1 cubanelle or green bell pepper, seeded and finely chopped

1 medium eggplant, cubed

6 ripe plum tomatoes, peeled, seeded, and finely chopped

1 tablespoon capers, rinsed well and drained

1 tablespoon golden raisins (preferably sultanas)

1 tablespoon pine nuts

⅛ teaspoon unrefined sea salt

¼ teaspoon freshly ground black pepper

DIRECTIONS

1 Preheat the oven to 425 degrees.

2 In a lightly oiled baking pan, place the fish. Bake until the flesh flakes easily, about 20 minutes. Keep checking for doneness.

3 In a large, wide skillet, warm 3 tablespoons olive oil over medium heat. Add the onion, celery, carrot, pepper, and eggplant, and cook until softer, about 6 minutes. Add the tomatoes, capers, raisins, pine nuts, salt, and pepper. Stir and cook until the sauce thickens, shaking the skillet, about 7 to 8 minutes.

4 Remove the fish from the oven, set in the sauce, allow to cook for 3 or 4 minutes, and serve.

PER SERVING: *Calories 323 (From Fat 120); Fat 13g (Saturated 2g); Cholesterol 51mg; Sodium 215mg; Carbohydrate 23g (Dietary Fiber 8g); Protein 30g.*

TIP: Use the freshest fish and produce you can find in this recipe.

NOTE: The sweet-and-sour notes of capers, raisins, and pine nuts are typical of Sicilian cuisine because the island was under Arab rule for five centuries.

VARY IT! Chicken also tastes great in this sauce. Vegetarians and vegans will appreciate the sauce (without the fish) on pasta or large couscous as well.

Frittata di Carciofi, Asparagi, e Cipolle Caramellate (Artichoke, Asparagus, and Caramelized Onion Frittata)

PREP TIME: ABOUT 15 MIN	COOK TIME: 45 MIN	YIELD: 6 SERVINGS

INGREDIENTS

¼ cup Amy Riolo Selections Extra-Virgin Olive Oil or other good-quality extra-virgin olive oil

2 medium yellow onions, very thinly sliced

1 pound baby artichokes, or frozen artichokes, thawed and drained

1 tablespoon lemon juice

1 bunch asparagus, trimmed and cut

1 bunch fresh basil or mint leaves, chopped

6 large eggs, beaten until foamy

¼ cup grated Pecorino Romano or Parmigiano-Reggiano cheese

¼ teaspoon unrefined sea salt

DIRECTIONS

1 Preheat the oven to 350 degrees.

2 In a large, wide, ovenproof skillet, warm the oil over medium-high heat. Add the onions and sauté, stirring occasionally, until softened and very dark golden in color, about 20 to 30 minutes.

3 Meanwhile, clean and trim the artichokes. Soak the artichokes in water to clean them. Drain and repeat until the water is clear. Peel away the outside leaves of the bottom half of the artichokes. Cut off the top quarter of the artichokes (at this point, the artichokes should look like flowers, and the tough, dark leaves should all be removed, leaving only the lighter-colored, tenderer leaves). If tough, dark green leaves remain, peel those as well. Fill a bowl with cold water and add the lemon juice; place each artichoke inside after it's trimmed to avoid discoloration.

4 Bring a large pot of water to a boil and add the cleaned artichokes. Return to a boil over high heat. Reduce the heat to medium-low and simmer until the artichokes are tender, about 15 to 20 minutes. Remove with a slotted spoon into a colander and drain.

(continued)

5 Bring the water back to a boil and add the asparagus. Reduce the heat to low for 1 or 2 minutes and cook until the asparagus is tender, about 1 minute. Remove with a slotted spoon and add to the skillet with the onions; brown for 4 minutes. Add the artichokes, and stir. Add the basil leaves, eggs, cheese, and salt. Mix well and reduce the heat to medium-low. Cook until the eggs are cooked through, about 4 to 5 minutes.

6 Put the skillet in the oven until the frittata top is golden, about 5 minutes. Cut into 6 pieces and serve.

PER SERVING: *Calories 269 (From Fat 138); Fat 15g (Saturated 4g); Cholesterol 215mg; Sodium 244mg; Carbohydrate 24g (Dietary Fiber 3g); Protein 11g.*

TIP: Use leftover vegetables or even spaghetti, as they do in Naples, in the frittata to get more variety and repurpose leftover food.

NOTE: *Frittata* is the singular Italian word for a baked omelet. *Frittate* is the plural form. Italians do not eat *frittate* for breakfast. The notion of eating eggs in the morning is unappealing to Italians, so it's usually part of a light dinner with salad, but you could eat it at lunch, too. If you were serving a frittata in a multi-course Italian lunch or dinner, it would be considered a main course.

VARY IT! Any vegetable you can think of tastes great in a frittata! Some people also use leftover egg whites or whole eggs to make their versions.

Cassola de Pisci a S'Ozzastrina (Sardinian Fish Stew)

PREP TIME: ABOUT 15 MIN	COOK TIME: 30 MIN	YIELD: 4 SERVINGS

INGREDIENTS

¼ cup Amy Riolo Selections Extra-Virgin Olive Oil or other good-quality extra-virgin olive oil

1 onion, finely chopped

2 cloves garlic, minced

3 red chile peppers, seeded and diced

1 tablespoon fresh oregano

1 cup fresh or canned reduced-sodium diced tomatoes

2 cups Homemade Seafood Stock (see recipe earlier in this chapter) or water

⅛ teaspoon unrefined sea salt

¼ teaspoon freshly ground black pepper

½ pound fresh clams (the smallest variety you can find)

1 pound grouper or other fish, whole

1 pound prawns or shrimp

2 tablespoons finely chopped fresh flat-leaf parsley, for garnish

DIRECTIONS

1 In a large stock pot, warm the olive oil over medium heat. Add the onion, garlic, chile peppers, and oregano, and cook for 2 to 3 minutes.

2 Stir in the tomatoes, stock or water, salt, and pepper, and bring to a boil over high heat. Reduce the heat to low and simmer, covered, for 20 minutes.

3 Stir, add in the clams, fish, and shrimp. Cover and cook until the clams are open completely, about 7 to 10 minutes. (Resist the urge to open and close the lid often, as this causes steam to escape, making it harder for clams to open and creating a firmer texture.) Discard any unopened clams.

4 Pour into individual cups or bowls, sprinkle with fresh parsley, and serve.

PER SERVING: *Calories 399 (From Fat 153); Fat 17g (Saturated 2g); Cholesterol 190mg; Sodium 306mg; Carbohydrate 14g (Dietary Fiber 2g); Protein 46g.*

TIP: Use the freshest seafood you can find — even if it's not the kind of seafood I list here.

NOTE: Sardinia is a Blue Zone island known for its productive and healthy contrarians. Dishes like this one help keep the locals going strong.

VARY IT! Use whatever seafood you like in this delicious preparation.

components of the
Mediterranean diet

» Making nutritious snacks, appetizers,
and desserts

» Discovering daily ways to add
sweetness to your life

Chapter 20

Fruit, Cheese, Nuts, and Desserts

RECIPES IN THIS CHAPTER

This chapter includes eight beloved Mediterranean dishes that beautifully exemplify the nutritious diet. Each recipe is versatile, relatively easy to make, and lesser known in the United States.

In this chapter, you discover the role that the particular recipes, ingredients, and dishes play in typical meals and get tips and tricks for enjoying them easily at home.

TIP

No meal in the Mediterranean region is complete without a hot drink at the end. Think of hot tea, espresso, or Greek and Turkish coffee as a period at the end of the sentence that is a meal. Many late-night meals are wrapped up with a digestif or an herbal tisane to help unwind after a long day.

What Traditional Mediterranean Desserts Really Look Like

For millennia, fruit and nuts were the original desserts. Originally sweetened with honey, rustic forms of cakelike pastries that we now associate with daily living were once reserved for offerings to the gods. The earliest recorded version of a birthday cake was a seasoned bun that the Ancient Egyptians would present to the pharaoh each year in honor of his birthday. At various times throughout history, grains, milling, and sugar were extremely expensive, so up until the late 19th and 20th centuries, those ingredients were still privileges enjoyed by royalty and the wealthy.

Nowadays, baking ingredients are readily available and inexpensive. Each Mediterranean country has its own rich tradition of dazzlingly beautiful and cloyingly sweet treats that are integral to holidays, special occasions, and weekly family meals and significant gatherings. It's worth a trip to the region just to witness and sample the pastry arts that are on display daily!

Despite the wide range of tempting options, local traditions when dining at home continue to conclude meals with fruits, cheeses, and nuts. From a health perspective, the great thing about this tradition is that it ensures you're getting plant-based foods and sometimes dairy in your daily diet. It also ends the meal on a slightly sweet note and cuts down on cravings for high-fat, high-calorie desserts.

Each country has its own customs regarding the serving of this final course, and they vary from place to place. Here are a few things that they have in common:

>> The freshest, seasonal fruit is always served.

>> The freshest, seasonal nuts help round out the course.

>> In France, Italy, and Spain, cheeses are also served with fruit at the end of a meal. In North Africa and the Levant, they are not.

>> Some French, Italian, and Spanish restaurants also include a cheese course among their dessert selections.

>> Throughout the region, it's typical to serve whole fruits on platters (such as figs, oranges, tangerines, and grapes) and nuts (still in their shells) on other platters.

>> Fruit, honey, spices, cheese, and nuts are also fashioned into simple desserts, as well as being incorporated into cakes and tarts.

Everyday versus holidays

The final or dessert course of the meal is based around the same principle as all other meals in the Mediterranean region. Daily meals eaten at home are delicious and varied but also healthful and balanced. Religious customs and fasting rituals still play a role in what people eat and when, even if it's so deeply interwoven into the culture that it isn't mentioned or discussed.

Many modern Italians no longer follow the rule of *fasting* (abstaining from meat) prior to taking communion at mass, but fish is still a Friday night special on Roman trattoria menus, and most Sunday dinners in Italy include meat (a tradition that started because people could eat meat after taking communion at mass on Sunday morning). Throughout the Mediterranean region, Fridays are the days of rest for Muslims, Saturdays for Jews, and Sundays for Christians.

Each weekly holiday is celebrated with a large gathering of family and/or friends, enjoying the best foods you can. Even in modern times, these weekly meals are comprised of more elaborate recipes (because the day off provides more time to cook), traditional dishes that are more rich and caloric in nature, foods that take time to be savored, and of course, elaborate desserts. In these cases, most of the pastries are purchased from outside. No matter where you are in the Mediterranean, there is no shortage of excellent pastry shops or bakeries. In fact, the ancient cities needed to have bakeries in order to be considered their own municipality. Nowadays, whether you're in Libya or Spain or Turkey, most neighborhoods have several bakeries to choose from.

Cultural attitudes behind desserts

Some families serve homemade baked goods for the holidays and weekly get-togethers, but it's very common to purchase them from outside. Until recently, kitchens, and especially ovens, weren't very reliable, so aside from a few beloved family recipes, many women (especially those who live in the city) didn't learn how or didn't have the option to bake inside the home. Communal ovens were used throughout the region to bake the daily bread. So, today, whether you're in Egypt or Israel or Italy, it's very common for families to purchase pastries for the holidays and special occasions.

When you receive an invitation to dinner or you're just going to visit someone, most people also purchase pastries or other baked goods to take as a hostess gift. Coffee and tea times are also important gathering occasions when pastries are served. In addition to pastry shops and bakeries (which specialize in bread and rustic sweets), in many Mediterranean countries, various communities are home to women who specialize in making specific desserts. Often they're called upon to make their own specialties. In Italy, many of the most cherished sweet recipes were passed down through the convents and sold as a way for the nuns to earn money for the church and charitable activities. In rural North Africa, a neighborhood might have a family that makes really great cookies, so they may purchase the sweets from them instead of from a shop.

Still, the idea of eating too many sweets is never promoted on a daily basis. Many people note the Mediterranean paradox of communities with great health where things like syrupy baklava and cream-filled pastries are commonplace. "Everything in moderation" is the only explanation for this phenomenon. When I post a picture of a tray of Mediterranean pastries on my social media feeds, that doesn't mean that I'm "cheating" on the Mediterranean diet. Those items are just as much a part of it as greens are; the only thing that's different are the amounts.

REMEMBER

According to the Mediterranean Diet Pyramid, the goal is to eat many plant-based foods daily — but sweets and desserts are still permitted sparingly, as is red meat. The notion of not having to cut anything out of your diet or your life is what has enabled the Mediterranean diet to be so effective and stand the test of time.

Mediterranean Fruit, Nut, Cheese, and Dessert Recipes

It's a stretch for me to consider pairing some of nature's most prized fruits with dairy and nuts and call them "recipes." The ideas in this section are so easy that they really do become second nature and a way of life. I like to consider them templates for ways to end meals on a sweet and nutritious Mediterranean note. Use them as guidelines and inspiration to create your own concepts!

The best thing about the recipes in this section is that they can fill in a lot of gaps in the modern diet and are really easy to implement. They can even be a quick breakfast on the run or a snack, or you can enjoy them when you have unexpected guests or as a light meal in lieu of fast food or the need to go to the supermarket.

Provençal Cheese Platter

INGREDIENTS

One 4-ounce wedge Camembert cheese

One 8-ounce log soft goat cheese

One 4-ounce wedge Roquefort cheese

¼ pound seedless red grapes, cut into clusters

1 cup plain almonds

8 thin slices French baguette (optional)

1 cup fresh herbs (such as basil leaves, lavender, mint, and so on)

DIRECTIONS

1 On a large platter or board, arrange the cheeses equal distances apart.

2 Fill in one space between the cheeses with grapes, another space with almonds, and the third space with the bread.

3 Decorate with herbs and serve.

PER SERVING: *Calories 566 (From Fat 406); Fat 45g (Saturated 19g); Cholesterol 72mg; Sodium 962mg; Carbohydrate 14g (Dietary Fiber 5g); Protein 30g.*

TIP: You can swap out your favorite French cheeses, such as Brie, Port Salut, and *Fromager d'Affinois* as well. It is nice to have a mixture of cheeses from different animal sources (sheep, goat, cow), as well as different aging levels.

NOTE: If you want to create this plate for one person, just use single serving portions of each item.

VARY IT! There are so many ways to change this up! You can swap out the three French cheeses with any other three cheeses from a Mediterranean country, and the board would still work. Add some Roasted Red Peppers (see Chapter 19) and olives, and this board can be transformed into an appetizer. Be sure to save extra leftover bits to use in snacks, sandwiches, or other recipes.

Calabrian-Style Figs with Ricotta and Honey

PREP TIME: ABOUT 10 MIN	COOK TIME: NONE	YIELD: 8 SERVINGS

INGREDIENTS

1 pint fresh figs

1 cup ricotta cheese, drained in a colander in the refrigerator overnight

¼ cup honey

1 cup chopped walnuts or almonds

DIRECTIONS

1 Wash the figs and make a cross about three-quarters of the way down from the stem with a paring knife.

2 Open the figs slightly and fill them with 1 teaspoon ricotta; set aside on a large platter.

3 Drizzle honey over the figs and sprinkle with nuts to serve.

PER SERVING: *Calories 214 (From Fat 115); Fat 13g (Saturated 3g); Cholesterol 16mg; Sodium 27mg; Carbohydrate 21g (Dietary Fiber 3g); Protein 8g.*

TIP: Chestnut and eucalyptus honey work best in this recipe.

TIP: This dish also makes a typical Southern Italian breakfast. It's my mother's favorite thing to eat!

NOTE: Ounce per ounce, figs have more nutrients than any other fruit. My ancestral homeland of Calabria, Italy is known for its prized varieties since antiquity, but excellent figs can also be found throughout the Mediterranean region and right here in the United States. Note that in Italy, ricotta is made from sheep and goat milk, not from cow milk. If you can find it, it would be a great ingredient to use!

VARY IT! You can also mix the honey into the ricotta and sprinkle the nuts on top like a dip for the figs. Or use Greek yogurt or goat cheese for the filling instead of the ricotta.

Egyptian Rice Pudding

INGREDIENTS

⅓ cup Egyptian rice, Calrose rice, Arborio rice, or short-grain rice

3¼ cups whole milk

1 cinnamon stick

Zest of 1 lemon

1 teaspoon vanilla

⅓ cup sugar

DIRECTIONS

1 Rinse the rice and drain well.

2 In a medium saucepan, add the milk, rice, cinnamon stick, lemon zest, vanilla, and sugar. Stir with a wooden spoon to combine and bring to a boil over medium–high heat.

3 When the mixture boils, after about 3 minutes, reduce the heat to low, stir, and cover.

4 Simmer for 1 hour and 30 minutes, stirring occasionally, until the rice is tender and liquid is absorbed.

5 Remove and discard the cinnamon stick. Allow the pudding to cool at room temperature. Then pour into a serving bowl. Serve, refrigerating any leftovers for up to 2 days.

PER SERVING: *Calories 163 (From Fat 39); Fat 4g (Saturated 2g); Cholesterol 13mg; Sodium 57mg; Carbohydrate 26g (Dietary Fiber 0g); Protein 5g.*

TIP: This creamy and satisfying pudding is also served at breakfast in North Africa and the Middle East.

NOTE: In Morocco, this style of pudding is stuffed into pastry sheets and formed in the shape of triangles, which are then fried and sprinkled with cinnamon and powdered sugar for special-occasion breakfasts.

VARY IT! Replace the rice with barley, farro, or your favorite grain of choice. Just be sure to adjust the cooking times to make sure that it's tender. You can use oat or almond milk instead of regular milk, if you want. To make a chocolate rice pudding, use ¼ cup Fair Trade cocoa powder and leave out the lemon zest.

Spanish Fruit, Nut, and Cheese Plate

| PREP TIME: ABOUT 10 MIN | COOK TIME: NONE | YIELD: 6 SERVINGS |

INGREDIENTS

1¼ pound wedge Manchego cheese

1¼ pound piece Cabrales cheese

One 2-ounce log goat cheese

1 cup Membrillo (quince paste cubes) or other preserves

1 cup Medjool dates

1 cup toasted walnuts

1 handful fresh strawberries or 1 bunch grapes

DIRECTIONS

1 On a large platter, arrange the cheeses equal distances apart.

2 Place the Membrillo, dates, and walnuts in small separate bowls or ramekins. Arrange the bowls in between the cheeses.

3 Arrange the strawberries or grapes around the openings on the platter.

PER SERVING: *Calories 1,097 (From Fat 665); Fat 74g (Saturated 44g); Cholesterol 176mg; Sodium 1,768mg; Carbohydrate 58g (Dietary Fiber 5g); Protein 55g.*

TIP: Delicious Spanish cheeses are becoming increasingly available in the United States. If you can't find them, substitute your favorites.

NOTE: To make this dish into an appetizer or serve it as part of an aperitif, add quality cured Spanish meats, olives, and roasted peppers to the plate, or create two separate ones.

VARY IT! In addition to strawberries and grapes, any seasonal fruit can be used on the platter.

Rose Water–Infused Fruit Salad

PREP TIME: ABOUT 5 MIN PLUS 5 HR TO OVERNIGHT FOR MARINATING	COOK TIME: NONE	YIELD: 4 SERVINGS

INGREDIENTS

1 cup cantaloupe, cubed

½ cup honeydew, cubed

½ cup watermelon, cubed

½ cup blueberries

½ cup sliced kiwi

¼ cup sugar

1 teaspoon rose water

¼ cup finely chopped fresh mint

DIRECTIONS

1 In a large salad bowl, combine the cantaloupe, honeydew, watermelon, blueberries, and kiwi.

2 In a small bowl, add the sugar, rose water, and mint, and mix together.

3 Drizzle the sugar mixture over the fruit and mix gently to combine.

4 Cover the bowl, and store in refrigerator for at least 5 hours or as long as overnight.

5 Transfer to individual bowls before serving.

PER SERVING: *Calories 99 (From Fat 3); Fat 0g (Saturated 0g); Cholesterol 0mg; Sodium 11mg; Carbohydrate 25g (Dietary Fiber 2g); Protein 1g.*

TIP: Always choose items that are in season to ensure the best flavor and nutritional benefit.

NOTE: Rose water is the essential oil pressed from non-chemically treated rose petals mixed with distilled water. A common element in Middle Eastern cooking since the 9th century, a little bit can go a long way. I love it splashed on watermelon and berries especially, but it's lovely in syrups, cookies, and puddings as well. Look for it in the baking or international aisle of your supermarket or buy it online or from a Middle Eastern or Indian market. If you can't find it anywhere, use lemon juice instead.

VARY IT! Mint and basil work well with most summer fruits, whereas thyme and rosemary work with roasted winter fruits. You can substitute rose water for lemon juice if you want.

Watermelon with Feta and Mint

PREP TIME: ABOUT 10 MIN	COOK TIME: NONE	YIELD: 8 SERVINGS

INGREDIENTS

4 cups watermelon cubes

1 bunch fresh mint, finely chopped

½ pound feta, cubed

2 tablespoons Amy Riolo Selections Extra-Virgin Olive Oil or other good-quality extra-virgin olive oil

DIRECTIONS

1 In a large bowl, place the watermelon, mint, and feta.

2 Drizzle with olive oil, stir, and serve.

PER SERVING: *Calories 132 (From Fat 86); Fat 10g (Saturated 5g); Cholesterol 25mg; Sodium 321mg; Carbohydrate 8g (Dietary Fiber 1g); Protein 5g.*

TIP: You can also make skewers out of this combination by threading pieces of watermelon with the feta cubes and mint leaves onto small wooden skewers. This is great for parties and entertaining!

NOTE: Only use sweet, seasonal watermelon in this classic Greek recipe, which is meant for summer.

VARY IT! Transform this delicious salad into a light meal by adding a cup of this mixture to cold quinoa and serving it over a bed of fresh greens such as arugula, spinach, kale, or purslane in the summer.

Date, Walnut, and Orange Torta

PREP TIME: 30 MIN	COOK TIME: 30 MIN	YIELD: 9 SERVINGS

INGREDIENTS

1¼ cup plus 1 teaspoon Amy Riolo Selections Extra-Virgin Olive Oil or other good-quality extra-virgin olive oil, divided

⅔ cup all-purpose flour or almond flour, plus extra for dusting pan

2 teaspoons baking powder

Grated zest and juice of 1 orange, separated

¼ teaspoon salt

4 large eggs, separated, divided

½ cup sugar

1 teaspoon vanilla

1 cup pitted Medjool dates soaked in water for 30 minutes, drained, and chopped

1 cup walnuts, toasted and chopped, divided

Powdered sugar, for garnish

DIRECTIONS

1 Preheat the oven to 350 degrees. Using 1 teaspoon olive oil, grease a 9-inch springform pan and dust it with flour.

2 In a small bowl, mix the flour, baking powder, orange zest, and salt.

3 In another bowl, beat the egg yolks and sugar together until thick and pale yellow, about 3 minutes. Slowly beat in the remaining ¼ cup of oil, the orange juice, and the vanilla. Stir in the flour mixture, then the dates and ½ cup of the walnuts.

4 Using clean beaters, in a separate bowl, beat the egg whites until stiff peaks form. Stir ⅓ of the egg whites into the batter; then carefully fold in the remaining egg whites until it looks like a cake batter but no white is visible.

5 Transfer the batter to the prepared pan. Place the pan in the center of the oven and bake until a toothpick inserted into center comes out clean, about 25 to 30 minutes.

6 Cool the cake in the pan on a rack. Place the cake on a platter and garnish with powdered sugar and the remaining ½ cup of walnuts before serving.

PER SERVING: *Calories 544 (From Fat 374); Fat 42g (Saturated 6g); Cholesterol 94mg; Sodium 206mg; Carbohydrate 41g (Dietary Fiber 3g); Protein 6g.*

TIP: The method in this recipe is a classic European-style one. The addition of olive oil gives it more flavor, better nutrition, and a moist texture.

NOTE: I always make two of these cakes at a time — one for myself and one to bring for hostess gifts. You can wrap them in plastic wrap and then aluminum foil after they're cooled and freeze them for up to a month. In Italy, a slice of this cake would be a great breakfast. It also works well with afternoon tea.

VARY IT! Swap out the dates for dried figs or apricots if desired. I also sometimes use crushed fennel or anise seeds as a flavoring instead of the orange juice and zest.

Apple, Almond, and Olive Oil Cake

PREP TIME: 30 MIN	COOK TIME: 45 MIN	YIELD: 10 SERVINGS

INGREDIENTS

⅓ cup plus 1 teaspoon Amy Riolo Selections Extra-Virgin Olive Oil or other good-quality extra-virgin olive oil, divided

¾ cup honey

3 large eggs

3 cups almond flour

¾ cup sugar

2 teaspoons pure cinnamon

1 teaspoon vanilla

4 large Golden Delicious (or favorite) apples, cored, peeled, and diced

1 tablespoon confectioners' sugar, for dusting

DIRECTIONS

1 Preheat the oven to 350 degrees. Grease a 10-inch springform cake pan with 1 teaspoon of the olive oil.

2 In a medium bowl, place the honey, the remaining ⅓ cup of oil, and the eggs, and mix to combine. Stir in the almond flour, mixing well to combine. Add the sugar, cinnamon, and vanilla, and mix well to combine. Stir in the apples.

3 Spoon the batter into the greased cake pan, spreading the mixture evenly and smoothing the top. Shake the pan to ensure that there are no gaps in the batter.

4 Bake on the center rack of the oven until a toothpick inserted in the center of the cake comes out clean, about 40 to 45 minutes.

5 Remove the cake from the oven and allow to cool to room temperature.

6 Remove the cake from the pan, dust with confectioners' sugar, and serve.

PER SERVING: *Calories 463 (From Fat 234); Fat 26g (Saturated 3g); Cholesterol 63mg; Sodium 23mg; Carbohydrate 55g (Dietary Fiber 5g); Protein 9g.*

TIP: Rustic, Italian farmhouse–style cakes like this one are great to have on hand for dessert, breakfast, or unexpected company. You can wrap it in plastic wrap and then aluminum foil after it's cooled and freeze for up to a month.

NOTE: If you're allergic to nuts, you can use all-purpose flour in this recipe instead.

VARY IT! Swap out any seasonal fruit for the apples in this recipe, depending on the season. For example, use cherries or berries in the spring, plum or peach slices in the summer, or pears in the winter.

6

The Part of Tens

Chapter **21**

Ten Easy Ways to Enjoy the Mediterranean Lifestyle Anywhere

Many of my students, readers, and followers tell me that they understand just how important the lifestyle choices of those living in the Mediterranean region are. "It's easy for them," they tell me. It's true that the Mediterranean region reinforces the lifestyle, and people living in those countries have it a little easier than those of us in other parts of the world. But that in no way prevents you from being able to achieve the same goals — sometimes even better ones — from abroad. Doing so just takes a little bit of extra work, planning, and inspiration in the beginning, but soon it becomes second nature!

Whenever I feel intimidated by the idea of doing something new, I remember the history of coffee in Yemen for motivation. When the Yemenis first obtained coffee plants from the Ethiopians, they were unable to grow them. Ethiopia's lush soil made it perfectly suited for coffee growing. Yemen, on the other hand, had dry, arid soil that was unable to produce good coffee crops. Over the years, though, the Yemenis developed very sophisticated irrigation methods in order to make the coffee grow the way it did in Ethiopia. Although it didn't happen overnight, eventually the coffee produced in Yemen became the most sought-after coffee in the world! The combination of local soil with the elaborate irrigation created chocolate-flavored notes in the coffee, and Yemen's port city of Al Makha became known for its coffee, which was coveted by Dutch traders.

The moral of the story: Not only is it possible to achieve great results with the Mediterranean lifestyle from abroad, but the extra effort will reward you in ways you can't even imagine. Not everyone who lives in a Mediterranean country practices these tenets — living in an area often makes people take things for granted. By mindfully making these practices a priority, you may have even greater results than someone who lives in the region.

In this chapter, I give you simple strategies to live your best Mediterranean-style life wherever you are!

Get Outdoors

Given the choice, most people in the Mediterranean would gladly choose to do anything outdoors instead of inside — from small tasks to major events. When Americans say they want to "get outdoors," they probably think of taking a trip to a nearby park or choosing to eat outside instead of inside during warm weather. But in Italy, Turkey, Greece, Egypt, Morocco, and many other places, it means much more than that. Morning coffee, afternoon tea, strolls after meals (especially dinner), a chat with a friend, drying laundry, reading, studying, and so on are all done outdoors.

Research shows that even ten minutes of outdoor exposure has positive effects on the psyche, mood, and brain power. Thirty minutes a day of fresh air, regardless of the weather, is said to be more powerful than antipsychotic medicine. For this reason, it's a great idea to make this practice a daily priority.

TIP

Here are a few ways to get more fresh air:

>> **Commit to going outdoors every day and despite the weather (with the exception of dangerous storms).** If you wait for a "perfect day," you cut down on your chances of going out. Bundle up in the winter, dress lightly in the warm weather, bring an umbrella for the rain, and plan accordingly. Just getting outside alone is enough.

>> **Practice an outdoor activity.** Gardening, fishing, grilling, walking, running, playing sports, and so on will ensure you spend more time in nature.

>> **Develop the habit of taking a *passeggiata* (a leisurely walk after dinner).** If your evenings are busy, try doing it after another meal, or whenever you like, daily.

>> **Volunteer for an outdoor activity such as chaperoning school events, coaching, cleaning up the ocean, and so on.**

These free, easy ways to getting outdoors will enhance your overall well-being (see Chapter 8). Best of all, many of them offer additional benefits, such as community building, physical exercise, and enjoying pleasurable activities that will make you feel better.

What about when it's really impossible to get outdoors? Bad weather, tight work deadlines, and sometimes even illness make it impossible for people to go outside. The next best thing is to increase outdoor exposure and *pretend* to be outside. By doing so — using guided imagery and your imagination — your body will actually begin to relax and feel the benefits of being outdoors, even though it isn't! Windows, courtyards, balconies, terraces, pictures, and sounds of nature can all help your mental and physical health.

TIP

Here are a few ways to get more outdoor exposure when you can't get outside:

>> **Pay attention to the outdoor exposure in your living space — windows, balconies, terraces, rooftops, porches, and so on.** Brainstorm ways to incorporate them more into your daily life. Can you eat or have coffee or tea on them? How about planting some herbs and flowers, reading, or studying there?

>> **Open your windows to let fresh air enter your home as much as possible.** In cold weather, even a little bit of fresh air in the morning will really help to change the energy in your home.

>> **Position your furniture so you're looking out windows instead of having your back to them.** That way, you can enjoy the outdoors more.

>> **Enjoy the sounds of nature.** If possible, open your windows to allow the sounds of birds in. If that isn't an option, listen to recordings of birds and other nature sounds, like the ocean. You can easily find them on the Internet — just search the web for "sounds of nature."

Spend Time with Friends and Family

Another common denominator of the Mediterranean lifestyle is the amount of time that people spend with friends and family. This is, in fact, one of the findings about the centenarians who live in Blue Zones and enjoy productive enjoyable lives well past a hundred years of age: They know that every day, at a certain time, they will sit down with loved ones at a table to eat a meal. You don't have to eat together, though — you can get the same benefit from sharing other activities.

The Blue Zones are five places around the world where people live longer and healthier than anywhere else. Two of the five — Sardinia, Italy, and Ikaria, Greece — are in the Mediterranean The others are Nicoya, Costa Rica; Okinawa, Japan; and Loma Linda, California.

Think about the everyday activities you do that you could share with another person. Perhaps it's walking, running, cooking, or shopping. It doesn't have to be a big event. In fact, it's better if you do the task often because that will help you to spend more time with others. Next, think about a set time at which you could do those things on a regular basis. Then ask a friend or family member if they would like to join you. If one person isn't always available, ask others in advance so you always have company.

Loneliness is a growing epidemic in the United States, so this seemingly "normal" idea may just be what we need to help people feel loved and cared for. Prior to the pandemic, three out of five Americans felt lonely. Men, young people, and those with new jobs seem to be affected the most. Luckily, loneliness is a problem you can solve easily and for free! With a little effort, you can foster better health not only for yourself, but also for your community.

Eat with Friends and Family

Eating communally, with friends and family, is the foundation of the Mediterranean way of life — you can't get too much of it. Chapter 4 discusses the benefits of and strategies for eating communally at length. But the basic idea is that you should find someone to eat with before deciding what to eat, just as the Greek philosopher Epicurus stated millennia ago.

Here are some tips:

>> Plan out who you're going to eat with on your calendar just as you plan out business meetings and doctors' appointments.

>> If you live in a home with others, try to enjoy at least one meal or eating experience together per day. Some families can't all be home for lunch or dinner, so a quick breakfast or late-night snack and weekend meals are good alternatives.

>> If you eat lunch at work, pick a lunch buddy to eat with.

>> When you can't help but be alone — for example, if you're working from home or self-isolating because of a pandemic — call or have a video call with family and friends while you eat.

Taking a few minutes every day to plan who you're going to eat with will have long-term payoffs for your physical and psychological health. You'll digest your food better, eat less, and absorb more of the nutrients from the foods you eat. Best of all, you'll enjoy yourself in the process, gain companionship, and reduce stress and the risk of loneliness.

Seek Out Hydrotherapy

Many healthcare professionals are now using the term the *blue effect* to describe the health benefits associated with being in the presence of water. The countries in the Mediterranean have access not only to the Mediterranean Sea itself, but also to many other seas, lakes, rivers, and other bodies of water. (Chapter 4 discusses the research behind this principle.)

TIP

Here are some easy and effective ways to enjoy the healing effects of water:

>> Write some water dates/activities down in your calendar at least a few times a week (or daily, if possible).

>> Go to a sauna and allow the steam to heal you. (Chapter 4 covers home saunas as well.)

>> Consider swimming and/or doing water aerobics for fitness.

>> Just looking at a body of water for ten minutes can do wonders for your health. It doesn't need to be an extravagant locale — a creek, stream, pond, or lake can do the trick.

Go Green

Just as the blue effect underlines and highlights the importance of water, the green effect proves just how important it is to be around greenery. Mother Nature created a great deal of nature with the color green — it's the only color that our eyes can look at without needing to adjust. Looking at green in nature has a calming effect on the psyche. (Turn to Chapter 8 for more information.)

Nature-deficit disorder was a term coined in 2018 to support the theory that children with attention deficit hyperactivity disorder (ADHD) focused better after being outdoors. Regardless of your age, the greener the outdoor access, the more your concentration will be improved. Natural light also helps people to heal faster. Hospital studies have shown that patients with a view of trees outside their windows recovered better than those staring at a brick wall, and when the additional benefit of fresh air is added in, the results are even better.

TIP

Here are some simple tips for getting more of the green into our lives:

>> If you're indoors, try to sit next to a window with greenery if possible.

>> Do as many of your activities outdoors if possible.

>> Take a walk in a park or the greenest area possible daily.

>> Bring green plants into your home, and plant trees in your yard, if you can.

>> Position your desk and any places where you do your daily work to face greenery if possible.

>> When choosing outdoor locations to spend time in, choose the greenest ones possible.

Make Something Meaningful

Doing work that is meaningful to you — whether it's a random daily act, a hobby, or your career — goes a long way toward promoting feelings of well-being, a sense of purpose, and something to look forward to. All three components are integral to mental and physical health. The art of looking for and assigning meaning to daily tasks is very important in the Mediterranean region. People take great pride in growing their own herbs, vegetables, and fruits when possible. They appreciate artisan work and handicrafts that are at the heart of their culture. They like the notion of connecting the past to the present and the future.

If you haven't done so in a while, set aside some time to consider what's meaningful to you in your life and in your work. How are you emulating or embodying those values on a daily basis? For example, you may have a job that you aren't so happy with, so a hobby or weekly activity that's pleasurable may give your life meaning. But what about the job itself? Is there a way to make it meaningful to you, even though you don't like the overall work? You may be able to find things you love even in less-than-ideal situations, and when you do, those situations usually transform themselves.

When I was young, for example, my mother gave me the "chore" of cooking for the family when she went to work. Although I loved baking and cooking with her and my grandmother, the notion of having to get a tasty and nutritious meal on the table each night with whatever ingredients she left me wasn't exciting to me. At that point, cooking did feel like a chore. A few weeks in, even though I was only 15 years old, I thought to myself, "I'm going to have to do this anyway, so what's the way that I can enjoy it the most?" I decided that the way I could find pleasure in my nightly task was by challenging myself to make the best dish possible out of what my mom left out for me. Two decades later, I had a career, a passion, and a meaningful life plan based around cooking. If you would've asked me what was meaningful to me when I was 15, I would've only thought of fashion, so the idea that I would find meaning in something that could've easily been dismissed as a meaningless chore is an example of how you can transform your life and your health by what you find meaningful.

TIP

Here are some ways to find more meaning in your daily life:

>> Make a list of what's meaningful to you, and do it as much as possible.

>> Examine your seemingly meaningless activities and try to assign a different meaning to them.

>> Understand that even meaningless tasks serve a purpose. Our brains work better when we do a combination of mundane work along with deep thinking.

>> Don't seek others' approval to validate what means the most to you. All that matters is what *you* value; the opinions of others don't matter.

Spend Time Doing What You Love or Nothing at All

This tip is a two-for-one: First, spend time doing what you love, and second, do nothing at all. Both are important, and both should be done on a daily basis. Chapter 7 discusses the numerous benefits of doing what you love. Whether it's work, play, sports, or volunteering, the activities that give you the most joy have a great impact on your health. There are obviously many things in life that you have no control over. But by choosing to purposely do what you love, you create positive emotions and, therefore, pleasure hormones that lift your spirit and calm your mind. Those good feelings translate into less stress and pain, as well as more enjoyment and good health. Your sense of security is also enhanced. Bottom line: Do more of what you love to do, as often as possible.

On the flip side of the coin, there is the Italian art of *dolce far niente* ("sweet doing nothing"), which is also practiced throughout the Mediterranean. The Italians, however, truly have kicked this tradition up a notch by naming it and proudly embracing the pauses they take in life in order to enjoy, literally, doing nothing. This doesn't happen by accident, and Italians are not lazy, nor have I ever heard of an Italian being bored. *La dolce far niente* is all about carving out that sweet spot in your day, week, month, or year when you can truly do nothing and feel good about it. You feel good because you know that you deserve it, and you know that it's good for you. You feel good because you know that when you return to work, your family, your friends, and your projects, they'll all benefit from the well-planned-out rest that you took.

TIP

Here are some ways to enjoy *la dolce far niente*:

>> Set aside a few minutes each day that are not planned. Bask in the sun, walk in the rain, sit back, and relax — if even just for a few minutes.

>> Plan a day (or as long as you can) every week, every month, or a few times a year when you can literally do nothing. Clear your schedule — don't accept any responsibilities or make any plans. When you get the urge to do something, let it be something relaxing and pleasurable.

Embrace Culinary Medicine

In the recipes in this book, I discuss ingredients that help the body to heal, keep illness at bay, and help people enjoy better, longer lives. The term *culinary medicine* refers to the art of cooking combined with the science of nutrition. Mediterranean cuisine, regardless of the particular country it originated in, fills the bill perfectly. People throughout the region turn to food time and time again to address health concerns and to stay fit.

TIP

In addition to the information earlier in this book, here are some suggestions:

>> **Make a list of any health concerns you have, and identify which foods, herbs, or spices are beneficial to the particular condition.** Make a meal plan using more of those foods.

>> **Adopt extra-virgin olive oil as your fat of choice.** Just a few tablespoons a day of good-quality extra-virgin olive oil will help reduce inflammation (which leads to all illness), coax more nutrients out of other foods, give the body omega-3 fatty acids, and keep many illnesses at bay.

>> **Make aromatics your friends.** Use garlic, onions, shallots, herbs, and spices as much as possible for their potent nutrients and flavor-enhancing properties without the fat or sodium.

>> **Plan a ritual involving herbal teas.** Discover which teas are best for your particular state and start by drinking at least one a night after dinner but up to three a day for maximum effect. I enjoy dandelion root for detoxing after winter, ginger for calming the stomach, and anise to help me sleep.

Eat Plenty of Fresh Fruits and Vegetables

You've probably heard the old adage "Eat the rainbow," and the advice is just as sage now as it was then. Planning your meals around fruits and vegetables, especially if they're in a variety of colors and locally grown, will play a part in your attaining maximum health.

The reason it's important to choose a variety of colors is because different color groups in produce usually offer different benefits.

Fruit makes an excellent snack or dessert. Green leafy vegetables should be the first choice every day, along with cruciferous vegetables. Make sure you're getting kale, spinach, purslane, arugula, collards, broccoli, Brussels sprouts, cauliflower, lettuce, and other healthful vegetables as often as possible.

Instead of planning meals around protein, such as chicken or fish, start by deciding which three vegetables you're going to cook with, and then add a bit of chicken or fish to them.

Be sure to drink a lot of water to help your body digest the fiber.

Make the Best Out of Any Situation

Last but definitely not least, learn to ride the waves, sing in the rain, and make the best of life. All Mediterranean countries, cultures, and people have had their own fair share of adversity. Older and indigenous cultural groups seem to be more grounded during times of strife than those in more "modern" societies. No one likes difficulty, but some people accept it as a part of life, let it go, and move on more easily than other people do. From a conceptual standpoint, people in places like Tunisia, Lebanon, Sicily, and Morocco have become generationally accustomed to looking beyond the perils of a particular moment to envision a brighter future ahead. In addition, millennia of converging cultures have taught them to look for the humor, the silver lining, the lesson, and the blessing in every situation.

There are two lovely expressions that I enjoy hearing often in Egypt. One is *alhumdullilah*, which means "Thank God"; the other is *ahsan*, which means "better" (meaning, "It's better like this"). Whenever you tell someone about a seemingly negative thing that happened to you, they'll immediately respond with *alhumdullilah* and/or *ahsan*. *Alhumdullilah* obviously shows gratitude. Even in seemingly negative situations, many Arabs and Muslims will give thanks, which assumes that God has an even better plan for them and that the apparent misfortune may just be a blessing in disguise. Next, they'll say *ahsan*, and they'll list the reasons why your mishap may just be a good thing. Then they'll often tell a joke to lift your spirits.

I'm sure Egyptians aren't the only people to say these things in this way, but it was in Egypt that I was first impressed by the profound impact that those words had on me personally, and also could be used as a way to pivot from a negative experience. Because pain is inevitable, having a formula to help you make peace during those times is crucial to your optimal health in the long run.

TIP

When you're experiencing something that seems negative, here are some ways to make the best of it:

» Take three deep breaths and acknowledge the fact that it may be the beginning of something better.

» Give thanks for whatever is happening and for a solution (even if you don't know what it is yet).

» Say "It's better this way because . . ." and then list any possible ways you can think of that it's going better.

» Give thanks for as much as possible in your life.

» Focus on things that you love and positive things that you can change.

» Know that even the worst times are only temporary, and seek comfort from friends, loved ones, and confidants.

Chapter **22**

Ten (or So) Creative Strategies for Communal Eating

Sharing meals is a way of life in the Mediterranean region, so much so that it's the base of the Mediterranean Diet Pyramid (see Chapter 13). Unfortunately, most people in the United States are missing out on this beneficial and tasty tradition. Most of us treat mealtimes as an afterthought — we grab breakfast on the go, inhale fast-food lunches at our desks, and squeeze in evening meals amid a flurry of activities. We're lucky if we find time to sit down for Sunday dinner or meet friends for a midweek coffee. But overall, communal eating is the exception, not the rule. The COVID-19 pandemic changed that slightly, for the better — many people around the world began reclaiming the joys of connecting at the table and of being together while eating.

Residents in Sardinia are ten times more likely to live past 100 than people in the United States. Researchers attribute their longevity to daily communal eating and the psychological security of being surrounded by loved ones. But every country and culture in the Mediterranean region has its own way of encouraging people to plan meals and eat together. This tradition also has been linked to improved digestion and eating less overall. Chapter 10 highlights the benefits of eating communally; this chapter shows you how to put it into practice.

First, Decide Who to Eat With

I'm sometimes asked, "If there is one person you could enjoy a meal with — from past or present — who would it be?" I usually answer that I would like to spend it with my grandparents (bless their souls), but then immediately remember that they, even in spirit form, are always present. I like to think that we never truly eat alone, because our ancestors are always with us. My dear friend and fellow cook-book author/TV host Jonathan Bardzik says that if you eat food from farms, you're never alone because the people who grew the foods are with you at the table.

REMEMBER

The table is a place that's built for connection. If there is one important takeaway from this book it's to remember to think about who you're going to eat with before thinking about what you'll eat. Yes, it requires a few steps of extra planning in the beginning, and there may be some practical, logistical obstacles to overcome, but it's well worth the effort. In addition to preventing loneliness, dining with other people provides psychological and physical benefits (see Chapter 10).

TIP

Think about who you'd most like to eat with. If those people are local, great. If they live with you, better yet. If they aren't, that's okay, too. Make a list of all the people you enjoy spending time over a meal with, and keep it handy the way you would a grocery list.

Review Your Schedule

After you've made a list of who you'd like to eat with, take a look at your schedule. You can do this on a daily, weekly, or monthly basis. It really doesn't matter how much time you spend planning, the important thing is to get into the habit of choosing who to eat with. When you find the times in your schedule that will allow you to eat with someone else, whether in person or virtually, make a note of it.

Next, contact the people on your list to see if they're available to eat at the same time. Let them know that you'd like to spend more time with them, and you're aware of the health benefits of doing so. Your loved ones will probably be thrilled at the idea!

Brainstorm

Think about ways in which it would be appropriate and practical to dine with the people on your list. Fine-dining restaurants and extravagant dinners, though wonderful, aren't the goal. Your mission is just to eat more meals with people you care about. It could be a salad or sandwich in the park, a Sunday brunch, a weekday breakfast, tea time, a picnic, a virtual call where you both have your food ready at the same time. . . . The important thing is the human contact and being able to look forward to spending a meal with someone.

Initially, while brainstorming, you may feel some of the stigma around eating communally. For example, many people associate eating a meal with someone of the opposite sex as a date. Others think that you have to be married, part of a couple, or a relative of someone to dine with them. Nothing could be farther from the truth — and as long as you're clear about your intentions, you don't have to worry about your intentions being misunderstood.

Whenever I happen to be traveling or dining alone somewhere in the Mediterranean region, the restaurant owner, a waiter, or a local resident will come and sit with me to keep me company. The Mediterranean approach of wanting to take care of others and accompany them through their meal is a good model to emulate.

There is also a lot of stigma attached to which meal we eat together. The Mediterranean lifestyle promotes large, communal lunches. But it doesn't have to be just lunch that you share. In the United States, we usually associate dinner with socialization, but you can bond just as easily over breakfast as you can over dinner. Busy couples and families are taking advantage of a communal breakfast (or other dining opportunities) to enjoy a bit of time together before their hectic days begin.

Join a Club

Supper clubs, book clubs, cooking clubs, and many other organizations include a meal as a part of their agenda. If you live alone or are just looking for other reasons to socialize and get more communal meals in, this is a great avenue. In addition to dining communally, these clubs will allow you to foster your passions and share them with other like-minded people. You'll be building the community, making new friends, and learning and engaging in meaningful activity, all at the same time. Best of all, the clubs have meetings at set times, so you can fit them easily into your schedule.

One of my dear colleagues is an amazing chef. He loves to cook, bake, and eat, and he's amazingly talented at those tasks. His wife, on the other hand, does not love food and eats only a very little bit. They have a wonderful marriage otherwise, so in order to foster his creativity, my friend started a supper club. He organizes weekly meals based on a different theme in his home each week. Attendees sign up for a certain number of spaces online and contribute a small amount toward expenses. My friend often solicits assistance from other guest chefs to create theme menus, which leads me to the next idea. . . .

Host Theme Parties

Some people refrain from entertaining because they believe that they have to have everything "ready" for whoever they're eating with, and busy schedules don't allow for prep work. If you can relate, keep in mind that working as a team can be fun and efficient. Assign one person the responsibility to pick up the groceries (or order them online), and cook together. It allows for more communal time in the kitchen.

Potlucks also make the perfect, easy-to-create theme parties. Decide on a theme and a place, and ask your friends to bring a dish. You can also switch up the locations — at different friends' houses, at parks, at work, and so on. The important benefit of theme parties is that they're fun and give people an excuse to get together. I often have theme-party cooking classes where we pick a menu from a different place in the Mediterranean. This helps my students learn more about the dishes and culture of a specific country.

In my personal life, I've also started doing theme dinners for every Sunday supper that I have in my home. I think about a place I would love to go back to and who I would like to share that experience with. Then I choose the music and the menu (sometimes elaborate, other times just one item). Next, I set the table in a way that reminds me of that place and the overall mood I want to create. I dress appropriately and stream videos from those places on the TV or a computer screen near the table. These dinners have become a fun and rewarding conclusion to my week, and a way to get motivated for the week ahead.

Be a Lunch Buddy

Many people have the most interaction with others during their workday, so lunchtime is a great time to eat together. Ask your coworkers to join you for your midday meal or invite a friend to lunch. With work lunches, just as with family dinners, it's important to set some ground rules in order to make them enjoyable and healthful. For example, agree not to "talk shop" at the table. Let your lunch be about light topics that you enjoy — a midday escape from the stress of work.

REMEMBER

Most Americans don't have very long lunch hours the way people in the Mediterranean do, so use whatever excuse you can to make lunch more pleasurable.

Enjoy Virtual Meals

If you can't eat with anyone, a virtual option is second best. When I'm working from home, writing and testing recipes, this option is the best for me. I can't invite people over, because my friends are all working or too far away to visit at lunchtime. Each morning, as I plan out my day, I decide who I'm going to call at lunchtime. I get to catch up with others while I enjoy lunch, and it gives me the emotional boost needed to finish my work.

One of the silver linings of the COVID-19 lockdown was everyone's newfound familiarity with and appreciation of video calling. I hope this trend continues for friends and family who live far away, because it really can be fun to feel so closely connected to those in distant places. Plus, scheduling a virtual meal takes some advance planning, so you're much more likely to follow through with it than if you just left your dining companion up to chance.

Volunteer

Many of my friends find that volunteering is a great way to not only give back to the community, but also make new acquaintances and even share common meals. Depending upon the setting, if you volunteer on a regular basis, eating together can become customary. One of my friends brings birthday meals in to a place where he volunteers for his colleagues' birthdays. My friends and I normally go to dinner after volunteering at an event. Many sports coaches I know enjoy a meal with their teams after a game. Regardless, it's all good for you, and it leads to the greater goal of increasing communal meals.

Commit to the One-Meal-a-Day Minimum

In a perfect world, we would eat all our meals communally, and everything would be set up to help us do that. In reality, however, things are different. Committing to eating just one meal a day communally — whether in person or virtually or a combination — is a huge act of self-respect, respect for others, and respect for your community. It doesn't matter what meal you choose or where you choose to eat it. Making this decision will put you on common ground with the residents of the Blue Zones (see Chapter 21) who live enjoyable, productive lives well into their hundreds. So, whether it's breakfast, lunch, dinner, afternoon tea, Sunday brunch, a picnic, or a party, take your pick and start planning!

Chapter **23**

Ten (or So) Fun Ways to Repurpose Food and Eliminate Waste

Repurposing food has always been a way of life in the Mediterranean region, where cooks are known for using leftovers in ingenious ways and doing everything in their power to reduce food waste. Just like indigenous people from around the globe have customarily used all the ingredients that nature provided them with, so do people in the Mediterranean region. To do otherwise is considered wasteful and disrespectful of both the environment and nature's bounty.

Eliminating waste and repurposing food are two trends that are on the rise in the United States and elsewhere. My hope is that they stay popular long after the press attention fades. We can save time, money, and the environment by maximizing the ingredients we have. Doing so also fuels our creativity and makes us feel more responsible. Here are some of my favorite ideas to reduce waste.

Make "Tutto Fa Brodo" a Way of Life

Tutto fa brodo means "Everything makes broth" in Italian, but the literal translation means "Every little bit counts," and it's a saying I utter on a daily basis. *Tutto fa brodo* is the Mediterranean way of being appreciative of everything we have. If you have enough little bits, after all, you can create something great. For example, you can come up with a great broth with little bits of leftover food.

TIP

I always start my Mediterranean diet classes by teaching how to make broth. You can find base recipes for it in Chapter 18, because making homemade broth saves not only money, but also a lot of unwanted calories and sodium (even reduced-sodium broth still has a lot of it). Plus, you'll get a much better-tasting and better-looking finished product. I save the tops of cut celery and carrots, onion peels, and leftover bits of herbs and tomatoes to make my vegetable stock. Shrimp shells are perfect for seafood stock, and roasted bones make a fantastic meat stock. If you make your own broth, your soups, stews, and sauces will sing with flavor, and your health will thank you for it!

Make Soups and Stews

When you've got homemade broth (if not, just use water), you can use your leftover grain of choice (rice, pasta, quinoa, barley, and so on) with leftover legumes or beans and vegetables to make a unique soup or stew. If you just have leftover stock and leftover vegetables on hand, you can puree the vegetables and add a little bit of stock to create a creamy soup as well.

Use Leftover Food for Sandwiches, Panini, and Shawarma

Anyone who's ever made a sandwich the day after Thanksgiving can attest to the fact that they're a great way to use leftovers. Combine your favorites creatively between two slices of fresh bread, and you're likely to have a combination that you like even better than the original meal! One of my favorites are the meatball sandwiches that we used to eat on Mondays when I was growing up. Most Calabrians make meatballs on Sunday as a second course. On Monday, the leftovers get repurposed by being sliced and placed between a sub-type roll and layered with provolone and/or mozzarella cheese and sauce. When heated, they become magically hard to resist! Hot, pressed sandwiches, like panini are also a great way to give new life to vegetables, chicken, and meat.

Shawarma is the thinly shaved rotisserie meat popular in the Middle East; it's known as gyro in Greece. In Egypt, I learned to make a skillet version by heating leftover shredded chicken with already sautéed onions, peppers, and tomatoes and a few spices. There, the mixture is topped with tahini and wrapped in pita with additional vegetables and pickles. You could also serve the same filling over rice or grains, or use it to stuff bread or in a wrap.

Puree Leftover Vegetables

Leftover vegetables often take on a new life when pureed. I add a little bit of water or stock to a blender, along with cooked or grilled vegetables, to come up with a puree. Then I taste it, season it, and decide if it would work best as a sauce or as a soup. If I decide to make it into a soup, I thin it out with more stock to make it thinner.

Another great way to use up the puree is to create what Italians call a *sformato* (a molded appetizer that consists of a puree with ingredients like pecorino or Parmigiano-Reggiano cheese, bits of vegetables, and/or meat stirred in). *Sformati* are spooned into greased ramekins and baked until set, usually 15 minutes at 400 degrees for small ramekins is enough. Leftover asparagus, corn, peppers, zucchini, cauliflower, carrots, and broccoli are all great *sformato* material.

Make Omelets, Frittatas, and Tortillas

One of the reasons why omelets are so popular on brunch menus is because they allow restaurants to repurpose leftover ingredients in them. You can do the same with Italian frittatas and Spanish tortillas as well. Potatoes, eggplant, zucchini, peppers, cheese, asparagus, artichokes, mushrooms, tomatoes, olives, spinach, kale, dandelion greens, purslane, arugula, beans, and legumes can all be incorporated into egg dishes to give them new life.

In Italy, it's also common to make frittatas out of leftover spaghetti. When you get the technique right, that humble dish becomes a masterpiece!

REMEMBER

Egg dishes are eaten at lunch and dinner in the Southern European part of the Mediterranean. Nutritionally speaking, the combination of eggs and vegetables is a winner, so feel free to confidently serve these dishes well beyond the traditional breakfast hours.

Toss It into Salads, Bowls, and Wraps

Although salads, bowls, and wraps are not traditionally Mediterranean in style (no one in the region sets out to make a large salad into a meal), they *are* good ways to use up leftovers and allow you to combine nutritious and authentic ingredients. For this idea, I suggest storing all your leftovers — whether they're meats, seafood, poultry, dairy, or vegetables — in clear containers and stacking them on a shelf in the fridge. Always have the same type of containers full of lettuce, a precooked bean or legume, and a precooked grain (such as quinoa, barley, farro, bulgur, or wheatberries), hard-boiled eggs, and pita on hand. That way, you can combine your leftovers into a salad, bowl, or wrap for a quick, easy, and nutritious lunch, dinner, or snack.

Make Your Own Croutons, Crostini, Bruschetta, and Tartines

Leftover bread has been used in a multitude of ways for millennia. Your croutons will have a lot more flavor and be better for you if you make them yourself. So will your breadcrumbs. Store them in the refrigerator for best use.

Bread is so sacred to the cultures of the Mediterranean that you'll still see people holding it to their lips and their forehead before throwing it out (if they need to do so as a complete last resort because it fell on the ground or was served in a restaurant). I'm one of those people. My cookbook mentor, Sheiilah Kaufman, actually wrote a book called *Upper Crusts,* all about repurposing bread. Sweet and savory bread puddings, strata, crostini, and bruschetta are just a few possibilities.

Bruschetta are much more widely used in Italy than they are in the United States, where they're limited to restaurants and the freezer section of supermarkets. In Italy, day-old bread is sliced somewhat thinly on the diagonal, drizzled with extra-virgin olive oil, and toasted on either side. Then it may be rubbed with a clove of fresh garlic and topped with any variety of ingredients, including tomato and cheese, cured meats, various cheeses, diced grilled vegetables, cured fish, and so on. The bruschetta are used as an appetizer in pizzeria and restaurants, as well as a snack and when entertaining guests. Leftover stewed cannellini beans are mashed with a fork and served on top of toasted bread with a drizzle of olive oil everywhere.

Another way to repurpose leftovers stylishly is with the French tartine tradition. Tartines are basically thin, open-faced sandwiches made out of toasted bread (usually wider, longer slices than the bruschetta). Think of your favorite avocado toast — this is a sort of tartine. You can use your imagination to combine leftover meats, vegetables, and cheeses with fresh produce and enjoy a tartine whenever the mood strikes. Creamy cheese, cucumber, and shrimp or smoked salmon is a classic. So is the combination of brie and/or cured meat with figs and a drizzle of honey.

Prepare Croquettes and Savory Cakes

Serving up your leftovers in the form of a croquette or savory cake will always leave your guests delighted and satisfied. Croquettes are popular throughout the Mediterranean region, especially in Spain, France, Italy, and Turkey. Leftover mashed potatoes, carrots, eggplant, zucchini? Stir in some grated Parmigiano-Reggiano or pecorino cheese, a handful of fresh herbs, and enough breadcrumbs to hold the mixture together. Shape it into balls, dip them into egg and more breadcrumbs, and fry until golden. Sicilians use leftover rice to make arancini, and Romans do the same to make croquette-shaped *supplí al telefono*. Leftover meat can be combined with Béchamel sauce, vegetables, and cheese to form croquettes as well. In Turkey, combining lentils, chickpeas, and beans with herbs is a popular way of making nutritious ingredients taste splurge-worthy.

Savory cakes are often made out of leftover rice, vegetables, and meats in the Mediterranean region. If you have a few cups of leftover rice, for example, you could layer it in a large buttered ramekin or baking dish (half of your rice needs to cover the entire bottom). Then layer leftover meat, cheese, and vegetables of your choice in the center. Add the remaining half of rice. Top with small pieces of butter or drizzle with olive oil and bake at 400 degrees until golden, about 20 minutes.

Incorporate Leftovers in Pasta and Rice Dishes

Italians rework leftovers into first-course triumphs of taste on a daily basis. That's how we're raised. Because pasta and risotto are generally the first course of lunch every day, it's important to serve them in different ways. By incorporating leftovers, you not only use up all your ingredients, but also get a unique first course as well. When making stuffed pastas, such as ravioli, tortellini, cannelloni, and others, it's very easy to use leftover cheeses, vegetables, or meat in the filling. My mind immediately drifts to the shredded, braised, leftover meat from a traditional Sunday meal being turned into a ravioli filling. Or a combination of small bits of cheese used as a tortellini filling. Leftover seafood makes a great filling, too!

And then there are *timballi*, the Sicilian baked pasta towers that are edible masterpieces. To make one of them, you can use a fluted pan, such as a Bundt pan or other round baking dish and layer pasta or rice dressed with sauce with the leftover ingredients that you have on hand (make sure the flavors go together), along with mozzarella, provolone, or other cheeses and perhaps some cubed leftover meat. Bake at 400 degrees until golden, about 30 to 45 minutes. Allow to set for a few minutes, and then, using a potholder, loosen the sides with a knife, and turn it out onto a plate to serve with more sauce and grated cheese. The same type of baked pasta dish as my Calabrian version — Pasta al Forno con Melanzane e Caciocavallo (Baked Pasta with Eggplant and Caciocavallo; see Chapter 19) — could also be made with a rectangular pan.

There are a multitude of ways that leftover ingredients can be used in making rice dishes. The first way is to toss the leftovers into the cooked rice to create a type of pilaf. This works especially well with long-grained rice like basmati. Fry some pine nuts or almonds and raisins in a bit of extra-virgin olive oil, and use as a garnish for the pilaf.

Italians make rice salads all summer long with boiled Arborio rice (cooked and drained as you would pasta) and then cooled. Then they toss it with diced meat and vegetables. You can use your leftovers as well as some legumes. This dish is eaten cold. When making risotto, you don't have to stick to the classic Milanese version. Just before adding your final bits of butter and cheese (after all the stock has been incorporated), you can just add in whatever leftovers you have in small pieces, and you'll have a new recipe to enjoy!

Appendix A
Metric Conversion Guide

Note: The recipes in this book weren't developed or tested using metric measurements. There may be some variation in quality when converting to metric units.

Common Abbreviations

Abbreviation(s)	What It Stands For
cm	Centimeter
C., c.	Cup
G, g	Gram
kg	Kilogram
L, l	Liter
lb.	Pound
mL, ml	Milliliter
oz.	Ounce
pt.	Pint
t., tsp.	Teaspoon
T., Tb., Tbsp.	Tablespoon

Volume

U.S. Units	Canadian Metric	Australian Metric
¼ teaspoon	1 milliliter	1 milliliter
½ teaspoon	2 milliliters	2 milliliters
1 teaspoon	5 milliliters	5 milliliters
1 tablespoon	15 milliliters	20 milliliters
¼ cup	50 milliliters	60 milliliters
⅓ cup	75 milliliters	80 milliliters
½ cup	125 milliliters	125 milliliters
⅔ cup	150 milliliters	170 milliliters
¾ cup	175 milliliters	190 milliliters
1 cup	250 milliliters	250 milliliters
1 quart	1 liter	1 liter
1½ quarts	1.5 liters	1.5 liters
2 quarts	2 liters	2 liters
2½ quarts	2.5 liters	2.5 liters
3 quarts	3 liters	3 liters
4 quarts (1 gallon)	4 liters	4 liters

Weight

U.S. Units	Canadian Metric	Australian Metric
1 ounce	30 grams	30 grams
2 ounces	55 grams	60 grams
3 ounces	85 grams	90 grams
4 ounces (¼ pound)	115 grams	125 grams
8 ounces (½ pound)	225 grams	225 grams
16 ounces (1 pound)	455 grams	500 grams (½ kilogram)

Length

Inches	Centimeters
0.5	1.5
1	2.5
2	5.0
3	7.5
4	10.0
5	12.5
6	15.0
7	17.5
8	20.5
9	23.0
10	25.5
11	28.0
12	30.5

Temperature (Degrees)

Fahrenheit	Celsius
32	0
212	100
250	120
275	140
300	150
325	160
350	180
375	190
400	200
425	220
450	230
475	240
500	260

Index

base recipes
  Braised Cannellini Beans, 233
  Chicken Stock, 237
  Dried Beans, 232
  Lentils, 234
  overview, 229–230
  Roasted Red Peppers, 231
  Seafood Stock, 236
  Vegetable Stock, 235
Bastianich, Lidia, 73
baths, benefits of, 53–54
bean dip, 171
bean salad, 171
bean skillet, 171
bean stew, 171
beans. *See also* legumes
  Braised Cannellini Beans recipe, 233
  Dried Beans recipe, 232
  Fresh Fava Beans with Asparagus and Poached
    Egg Salad recipe, 217–218
  quick meals containing, 171
  stocking pantry with, 162–163
Beets with Cinnamon Salad recipe, 219
beghrir, 192
behavioral activation, 72
bell peppers
  Roasted Red Peppers recipe, 231
  using as aromatics in recipes, 136
belly dancing, benefits of, 52–53
bicycling, as exercise, 78
Bileela (Creamy Wheatberry Cereal) recipe, 203
biodiversity, 163
blue effect, 269
Blue Zones, 69, 268
bocadillos, 193
boreks, 143
Bosnia, culture in, 109
bougatsa, 191
Braised Cannellini Beans recipe, 233
bravas-style seasoning recipe, 140

bread
  lavash, 144
  repurposing, 284–285
  Rustic Moroccan Barley Bread recipe, 200–202
breadcrumbs, 284
breakfast
  deciding on large or light, 154–155
  grab-and-go options for, 194
  overview, 189
  personalizing, 193–194
  recipes
    Bileela, 203
    Egyptian Fuul Medammes with Tahini, 199
    Green Shakshouka, 205
    Halloumi Mashwi bil Baid, 204
    Homemade Labneh Cheese, 195
    overview, 194
    Pan di Spagna, 198–199
    Rustic Moroccan Barley Bread, 200–202
    Spanakopita, 196–197
  sample menu, 155
  throughout Mediterranean, 190–193
Broccoli Rabe with Garlic, Extra-Virgin Olive Oil,
  and Chilies recipe, 222
broth
  Chicken Stock recipe, 237
  homemade compared to store-bought, 282
  Seafood Stock recipe, 236
  Vegetable Stock recipe, 235
bruschetta, 284
bulgur grain, 171
bulgur soup, 172

C
café, 193
café con leche, 193
cakes
  Apple, Almond, and Olive Oil Cake recipe, 262
  Pan di Spagna recipe, 198–199
  savory, 285

About the Author

As an award-winning, best-selling, author, chef, and television personality, **Amy Riolo** is one of the world's foremost authorities on the Mediterranean lifestyle. She is internationally recognized for sharing history, culture, and nutrition through her writing, programs, TV shows, events, products, and tours. A graduate of Cornell University, in 2019, she launched Amy Riolo Selections, her private-label collection of premium Italian imported foods. Amy makes frequent appearances on numerous television and radio programs in the United States and abroad. She is a chef and instructor for Italian Sensory Experience, with which she leads tours in Italy; she also leads tours with Indigo Gazelle Tours in Morocco and Greece. Amy's print work has appeared in *USA Today, Cooking Light, The Washington Post,* CNN.com, *The Wall Street Journal, Parade, Gulf News, The Jerusalem Post Magazine, Popular Anthropology Magazine, Ambassador, The Examiner,* and *The UAE National,* as well as hundreds of other national and international newspapers and magazines.

Amy released the second edition of her award-winning, best-selling *Mediterranean Diabetes Cookbook* (American Diabetes Association) in 2019. She has written multiple books with the American Diabetes Association and was the national spokesperson for their 2018 release, *Quick Diabetic Recipes For Dummies.* In 2018, Amy also released *Creating a Cookbook: How to Write, Publish, and Promote Your Culinary Philosophy* on Amazon. Her seventh book, *The Italian Diabetes Cookbook* (American Diabetes Association), was released in 2016, and was the number-one new release on Amazon.com. In 2015, she released *The Ultimate Mediterranean Diet Cookbook,* which was named one of the best Mediterranean diet cookbooks for 2021. Her third book, *The Mediterranean Diabetes Cookbook* (American Diabetes Association) was released in 2010; it received a starred *Publisher's Weekly* review, won the 2011 Nautilus Book Award, and was named "Best. Diabetes. Cookbook. Ever" by DiabetesMine.com. Amy's second book, *Nile Style: Egyptian Cuisine and Culture* (Hippocrene Books), won the World Gourmand Award for "Best Arab Cuisine Book" in the United States and was just released in a second edition. Her first book, *Arabian Delights: Recipes & Princely Entertaining Ideas from the Arabian Peninsula* (Capital Books), was chosen one of the "16 Volumes Worth Staining" by *The Washington Post.* She has contributed to, edited, and coauthored several other books and encyclopedias as well.

Dedication

To the memory of my nonna, Angela Magnone Foti, for showing me that food is the foundation upon which our families, communities, cultures, and lives are built upon; to my parents, for fostering my life's purpose; to my relatives in Crotone, Italy, who inspired me to promote our culture and traditions from the very beginning; and to everyone who strives to preserve the invaluable resources that the Mediterranean lifestyle has to offer.

Author's Acknowledgments

I owe my ability to write and promote the Mediterranean lifestyle strictly to destiny. Had I been born into another family or culture and not had the opportunity to live, work, and travel throughout the Mediterranean region, it would never have been possible. After decades of witnessing not only my own family, but people throughout the region, living and eating with both pleasure and health, I am convinced, now more than ever, that this is a goal that we can all achieve.

Destiny is also to thank for enabling me to get to know so many people and places in the Mediterranean and at such an intimate level. I believe that it truly "takes a village" to make a good chef and a good writer — and in my case, that village is a global one. I am honored and proud to say that I have learned from amazing cooks in places that I never dreamed I would even visit. To all of you who have shared a kitchen or a meal with me, thank you.

My nonna, Angela Magnone Foti, taught me to cook and bake, as well as valuable lessons that served me outside the kitchen. Because of her and our heritage, my first tastes of "Italian food" were Calabrian. Those edible time capsules formed a culinary bloodline between us and our relatives in Southern Italy. Because of her, I am able to prepare many of the same dishes that my Italian relatives do, even though I am a fourth-generation American. Nonna Angela gave me my first cookbook and showed me how cooking was not a mundane chore, but a form of magic that could unite people across distances and time. I owe my career to her and would give anything to be able to share more time in the kitchen with her. Cooking was so important to her that a few weeks before she passed, at 91 years old, she refused to go into the hospital because it was Christmastime and she told the doctors that she needed to be home so that she could "make cookies with Amy." It is an honor for me to be able to pass her knowledge on to my readers.

My Yia Yia, Mary Michos Riolo, shared her beloved Greek traditions with me, and I am happy to say that they have become woven into my culinary fabric as well — especially because many Italian regions were Greek colonies in antiquity. My earliest memories of cooking were with my mother, Faith Riolo, who would sit me on the counter and roll more meatballs and cookies than I could count. She taught me that food was not just something we eat to nourish ourselves, but an edible gift that could be given to express love. I owe my love of food history and anthropology to my father, Rick Riolo, for planting the desire to answer the question, "I wonder how they eat . . ." in my mind since childhood. It's a type of culinary curiosity that is never completely satisfied and gives me the motivation to continue my work each day. To my beloved little brother, Jeremy, you are my why, and I am grateful to be able to pass our family's knowledge down to you.

I would probably never have published a cookbook if it weren't for my mentor, Sheilah Kaufman, who patiently taught me much more than I ever planned on learning. I am proud to pass her knowledge on to others. I am very thankful to Chef Luigi Diotaiuti, for always believing in me and for encouraging me to foster my culinary medicine interests. I am also very grateful for the presence of Dr. Sam Pappas in my career. In addition to appreciating and supporting my work, he continues to collaborate on many of my health-related endeavors.

In Italy, I thank my cousins Franco Riolo and his lovely wife Pina; Tonia Riolo; my beautiful cousin, Serena Riolo, who I love cooking and attending culinary events with; and her brother, Vincenzo Riolo, for the bond and memories that we share; as well as my dear cousin Angela Riolo, for sharing my passion and continuously supplying me with authentic Calabrian recipes. In fact, I am immensely grateful to each of my *Cugini Calabresi,* as I affectionately call them. I am very grateful for their acceptance of me — as a third cousin — who they met later in life but embrace me wholeheartedly as someone who they grew up with. The sense of peace, happiness, and joy that I feel when we are together is second to none.

To my Italian Sensory Experience partners, Antonio Iuliano and Francesco Giovanelli, thank you for making my culinary dreams come true. I am also very grateful to Stefano Ferrari, owner of LIFeSTYLE and Cibo Divino, for importing and distributing my private-label products, along with Vince Di Piazza of DITALIA Fine Italian Imports for distributing them. Additional thanks go to Stellina Pizzeria, The Mediterranean Way, Milan Milan in Bermuda, Tastings Gourmet in Annapolis, and all the other retailers who carry my products. *Grazie mille* to Tommaso Masciantonio, Alessandro Anfosso, and Acetaia Castelli for partnering with me.

There is not a day that passes that I don't thank my close friend and business partner Alex Safos of Indigo Gazelle Tours for his support and collaborations. Alex has added beauty and depth to each of my days by enabling me to lead culturally oriented culinary tours in what have become my favorite places on the planet. In addition, he has enabled me to find my greatest joy in life: to learn and teach at the same time.

Throughout recent years I have been fortunate to be able to call upon the assistance of many dear friends who I love like family. Time and time again they have supported me and my projects in an amazing fashion. My beautiful and talented *sorellina,* Lisa Comento; #TeamAmy founder and marketing diva Gail Broeckel; the great chef, Paul Kolze; my favorite molecular gastronomist, Edward Donnelly; the multitalented Stuart Hershey; my friend and kindred spirit, Kim Lee; the five-star rock-star chef, Sedrick Crawley; and our newest recruit, Certified Executive Chef and Chief Master Sargent Jeff Fritz. I would also like to give a heartfelt thanks to my fantastic producer, Bradley Lewis, for being a great mentor and coach. To my Fairy God Sister, Kim Foley, you are the best.

I would also like to thank Dr. John Rosa for recognizing my contributions to the field of culinary medicine and for all the wonderful avenues of collaboration. To Marc Levin, President and CEO of the Maryland University of Integrative Health, thank you very much for the opportunity to work with such an important establishment. I am also very appreciative of my alma maters, Cornell University and Montgomery College, for recognizing my achievements.

At Wiley, I would like to thank Tracy Boggier for being so enthusiastic and great to work with. I truly appreciate the expert and efficient editorial support and guidance of Elizabeth Kuball, and thank Kristie Pyles for all her support as well. Wendy Jo Peterson and Grace Geri Goodale, thank you for your terrific photography, synergy, and overall appreciation of everything Mediterranean. Many thanks to the American Diabetes Association for introducing me to Wiley years ago.

I am forever indebted to Dr. Norton Fishman for diagnosing me and creating a team of doctors to enable me to heal. To my dear friend and sister, Kathleen Ammalee Rogers, I would not be here if it weren't for your care, support, and friendship, and I am always thankful to you for my health, career, and overall well-being. I am also forever grateful to Dr. Beth Tedesco and Dr. Mary Lee Esty, for enabling me to overcome my own illness and fulfill my dreams. My dear friend Susan Simonet is a constant source of guidance and inspiration. I have dubbed the amazing Monica Bhide "Leading Light" because she is a faithful and trusted friend who always brightens my days. To my trusted friend and colleague Jonathan Bardzik, thank you for helping me create joy daily. And finally, I would like to thank you, the reader, for joining me on this journey into an enjoyable and rewarding way of life.

Publisher's Acknowledgments

Senior Acquisitions Editor: Tracy Boggier

Project Editor: Elizabeth Kuball

Copy Editor: Elizabeth Kuball

Technical Editor: Sam Pappas, MD

Recipe Tester: Rachel Nix, RD

Nutrition Analyst: Rachel Nix, RD

Production Editor: Mohammed Zafar Ali

Photographers: Wendy Jo Peterson and Grace Geri Goodale

Cover Image: © Photo by Alex Safos, Owner, Indigo Gazelle Tours